Chasing the Surge

Life as a Travel Nurse in a Global Pandemic

by
Grover Nicodemus Street, R.N.

with
Sandra de Abreu Guidry-Street, M.D.
and
Ja-ne de Abreu

Copyright © 2021, JMFDEA Press

All rights reserved. No part of this publication may be reproduced, distributed, or transmitted in any form or by any means, including photocopying, recording, or other electronic or mechanical methods, without the prior written permission of the publisher, except in the case of brief quotations embodied in critical reviews and certain other noncommercial uses permitted by copyright law. For permission requests, write to the publisher, addressed "Attention: Permissions Coordinator," at the address below.

P.O. Box 235737 Honolulu, HI 96823

Ordering information: www.jmfdeapress.com

Printed in the United States of America

ISBN Hardcover: 978-1-7362954-3-4
ISBN Paperback: 978-1-7362954-5-8

First Edition

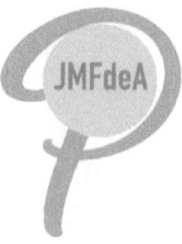

To all those in healthcare who work tirelessly, no matter the personal struggles and sacrifices to help save lives in these extraordinary times. And to every single person on the planet—for we have all been greatly affected by the COVID-19 pandemic. May we grow wiser as we learn from our challenges.

From our initial conversations about the idea of this book at Christmas to actually publishing it took four short months. It was incredible how quickly this came together. I provided the creative landscape and detailed stories in my voice, Sandra smoothed it out and added more medical research. Ja-ne crafted the structure and helped with ingenious editing and publishing. My family worked to make this come together as fast as humanly possible. I feel it was successful because we worked with a unique synergistic approach towards a common goal. We were united in the mission to help others in this pandemic.

To my wife, Sandra—thank you for putting up with my travels, being away from you for so long, and for interpreting my 'Nic Speak' (as you and Ja-ne call it).

Ja-ne Malafaia Francioni de Abreu, my favorite sister-in-law as co-conspirator. You were incredible to work with and I owe you my gratitude for making this project come to fruition.

Elise Guidry, Jacob and Hallie Guidry, Logan and Kaitlyn Guidry, our adult kids who helped with technical writing and proofreading; your input was invaluable to refine certain passages and to improve the flow of my ideas.

And to all the other beta readers who took time to read this manuscript and share their comments; I took everything to heart considering each and everyone's particular lens and how it would impact readers in those specific groups. "Walk a mile in their shoes," as the saying goes.

Thank you to the families and patients who shared their very personal stories at the end of this book. Your poignant words telling all of what you and your family went through in this crisis will positively affect someone's life.

Thank you, Sue Toth, for your patience and help in editing this manuscript. The sheer speed this came together and all the questions we threw at you must have been a whirlwind.

I want to take this opportunity to say this book is not intended to be a polarized political stance. I have never been one to stand on any soap box. It is an account of my tremendous experience as I navigated the uncharted waters of this COVID pandemic. Along the way, there were numerous obstacles and challenges I personally encountered in addition to the horrific suffering and death we as healthcare workers faced every day.

I hope you enjoy learning a little bit about COVID-19 and what went on behind the closed doors of hospitals as we cared for the sick in this crisis. Some of the names and locations were changed to maintain patient privacy, but the essential aspects of the situations are all true. It is incredible to think this could happen in a lifetime, but more unbelievably, these events happened in one short year.

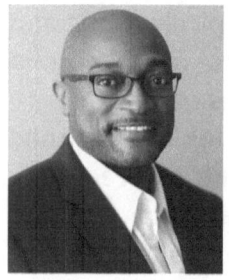

Grover Nicodemus Street has a BS in Nursing and a MBA in Healthcare Administration and Leadership. In the beginning of his career, he served as a Trauma Nurse in the US Air Force for 6 years and worked as a clinical instructor for 4 years. For 23 years, he has worked all over the USA as a trauma nurse, mostly in emergency departments and various intensive care units. Grover also has a fourth degree black belt in Taekwondo and black belts in Shotokan and Ishinryu. His inspiration for writing Chasing the Surge was to dispel widespread misbeliefs about the COVID-19 pandemic and to share his real experiences behind closed doors in hospitals. He felt compelled to especially help minorities understand more about this disease and also to learn about the science behind the vaccine as well as its safety.

COVID-19 Pandemic Timeline for USA

January 8, 2020

The Centers for Disease Control and Prevention (CDC) is closely monitoring a reported cluster of pneumonia of unknown etiology (PUE) with possible epidemiologic links to a large wholesale fish and live animal market in Wuhan City, Hubei Province, China. An outbreak investigation by local officials is ongoing in China; the World Health Organization (WHO) is the lead international public health agency. Currently, there are no known U.S. cases nor have cases been reported in countries other than China. —CDC Health Alert Network

January 9, 2020

Fifty-nine cases reported in China. Chinese authorities reported in the media that the cause of this viral pneumonia was initially identified as a new type of coronavirus, which is different than any other human coronavirus so far. Coronaviruses are a large family of respiratory viruses that can cause diseases ranging from the common cold to the Middle-East Respiratory Syndrome (MERS) and the Severe Acute Respiratory Syndrome (SARS). From the currently available information, preliminary investigation suggests that there is no significant human-to-human transmission and no infections among health care workers have occurred. —World Health Organization

January 10, 2020

Currently, there are no cases outside of Wuhan City. WHO does not recommend any specific health measures for travelers. International traffic—no restrictions recommended.

January 21, 2020

First US confirmed case of COVID-19. Patient returned from Wuhan on January 15.
 More than 200 cases confirmed in China. Four dead.
 Zhong Nanshan, MD confirms human to human transmission.

January 22, 2020

"We have it totally under control. It is one person coming in from China, and we have it under control. It's going to be just fine." —US President Donald J. Trump interview with CNBC

January 23, 2020

"Make no mistake. This is an emergency in China, but it has not yet become a global health emergency." — President Trump tweet
 300 additional infections in China. Thirteen additional deaths. The city of Wuhan is closed.

January 24, 2020

"China has been working very hard to contain the Coronavirus. The United States greatly appreciates their efforts and transparency. It will all work out well. In particular, on behalf of the American people, I want to thank President Xi!" —President Trump tweet

January 29, 2020

The White House announces the formation of a coronavirus task force to be led by Health and Human Services Secretary Alex Azar. —White House announcement

January 31, 2020

With over 9800 cases and over 200 deaths globally, WHO announces a public health emergency.

The secretary of the US Department of Health and Human Services, Alex Azar, declares a public health emergency. "While this virus poses a serious public health threat, the risk to the American public remains low at this time, and we are working to keep this risk low," Azar says.

	COVID CASES		COVID DEATHS	
JAN	Global 12,308	US 1	Global 265	US 0

February 2, 2020

"We pretty much shut it down coming in from China." —President Trump in interview with Sean Hannity

Global air travel is restricted.

February 3, 2020

US announces a public health emergency.

February 10, 2020

"Looks like by April, you know, in theory, when it gets a little warmer, it miraculously goes away…But we are doing great in our country…I think it's going to all work out fine." —President Trump at campaign rally in Manchester, NH

COVID death toll of 908 exceeds those of previous SARS crisis of 774.

February 13, 2020

"In our country, we only have, basically, twelve cases, and most of those people are recovering and some cases fully recovered. So it's actually less." — President Trump interview with Geraldo Rivera

February 17, 2020

Dr. Fauci doesn't want people to worry about coronavirus, the danger of which is "just minuscule." But he does want them to take precautions against the "influenza outbreak, which is having its second wave."—USA Today

February 24, 2020

"This Coronavirus is very much under control in the USA. We are in contact with everyone and all relevant countries. CDC & World Health have been working hard and very smart. Stock market starting to look very good to me!" —President Trump tweet

February 25, 2020

CDC warns COVID-19 meets two of three factors towards pandemic status.

February 28, 2020

WHO raises the global risk of coronavirus from high to very high.

February 29, 2020

"Right now at this moment there is no need to change anything that you are doing on a day by day basis. Right now the risk is still low, but this could change." —Dr. Fauci on The Today Show

	COVID CASES		COVID DEATHS	
JAN	Global 12,308	US 1	Global 265	US 0
FEB	Global 86,471	US 60	Global 2,978	US 0

TABLE OF CONTENTS

NEW JERSEY / 3

COLORADO / 37

NEW YORK / 53

COLORADO / 89

FLORIDA / 101

COLORADO /135

CALIFORNIA / 143

COLORADO / 171

CALIFORNIA / 175

COLORADO / 197

CALIFORNIA / 209

OTHER STORIES / 227

SOURCES / 257

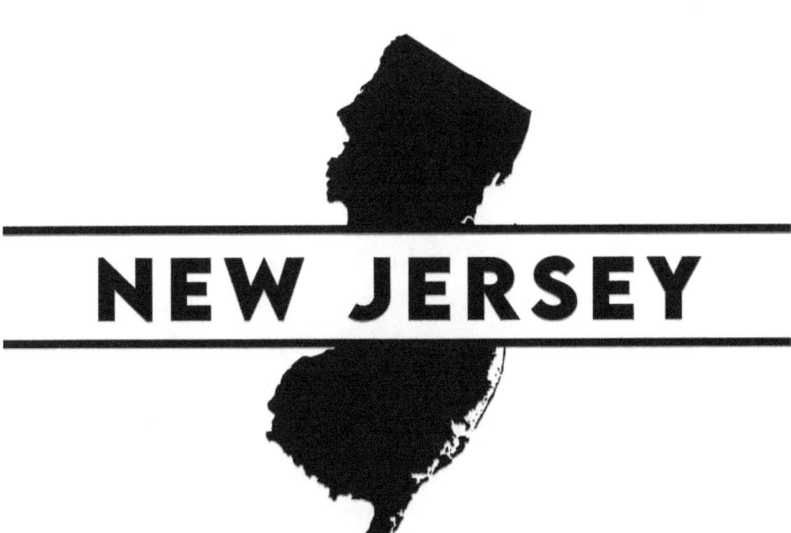

March 2, 2020

A tall Korean patient came into the emergency room with typical flu-like symptoms of fever over 103°F, body aches, vomiting, and a sore throat. He was pale and diaphoretic. I immediately gave him a mask and proceeded to get more information from him. The man reported he just returned from a trip to China two weeks ago, then gradually started feeling bad.

As a travel nurse working triage and Fast Track, it was my job to determine which area of the emergency department would be best suited to treat this guy. I would have put him in the main emergency room, but they were full up and had over fifty patients waiting to be seen. Fast Track had no extra beds, and twenty patients were waiting, but eventually I got him into bay #3. We tested him for influenza, which came back negative. Springtime is when hospitals usually see a lot of influenza and every year there are always some false negative tests. This patient was exhibiting typical flu symptoms, like most of the people coming in today. They all seemed to be in bad shape, being very short of breath and needing IV fluids and medications, which was a bit unusual.

The ED doc treated him with normal saline and Tylenol and sent him home with Tamiflu. Some patients came from New York hospitals to New Jersey because the expected wait there was at least twelve hours or more. Here it looked like it would only be about eight before getting to see a doc. It was looking like this flu season was going to be quite hectic.

March 4, 2020

I saw the Korean man from two days ago on a gurney in the hallway. Even though he was wearing a mask, I recognized him as I walked by. Maybe it was the flicker of the florescent lights, but the poor guy looked even more pale than last time. Pearls of sweat dotted his forehead and his skin had a sheen resembling wet dolphin flesh. Even though he wasn't my patient today, I felt compelled to stop.

"Man, you don't look so good. What's going on?" I asked.

He responded, "I feel horrible and I'm getting worse every hour. That medicine didn't work. They said the hospital is full, so I have to wait here."

"Yeah, we're busier than usual this week, like super busy. Stay strong and get better soon. I gotta get back to my station," I said and headed to the trauma bay.

Most ERs are divided into sections that concentrate categories of patients into smaller defined spaces. There is the Fast Track area for minor issues like colds or low-level injuries. A different area is for moderately ill patients with "walking pneumonia," dehydration, or other conditions needing treatment. These patients are usually stable enough to go home afterward. The area where I feel mostly in my zone is the trauma bay. It has the best equipment loaded with all the bells and whistles you would see on any ER show on TV. Patients coming in from bad car accidents to gun-shot wounds, stabbings to heart attacks, or strokes—they all come here. You name it, we can treat it.

Over the past couple of days, the ER was filling up with patients coughing, short of breath with fever and chills. Some had abdominal pain as well. The media was talking about this mysterious new viral infection in China that had already started to spread in Europe. There were a few cases in Washington state on the west coast that seemed to have started from passengers of cruise ships. They all were quarantined, so there was no way these patients coming in right now could be sick with this new coronavirus. We didn't even have a test here yet to check.

I think there was a disconnect between the reports from WHO and CDC compared to the messages we were getting from our government. Although we were busy, it wasn't like the hordes of patients as they suggested. The White House told us not to worry about the new infection. It was limited to a handful of patients and contained. Maybe this new virus was going to be like all other flu-like illnesses over the past years that started in China and never spread to the US to any great degree.

At the end of my shift, I got a call from the occupational medicine doctor. "How long were you with that patient the other day? You know, the one that just came from China," he asked.

"Probably ten minutes or so. Why?" I answered.

"How close were you standing to the patient? Was it two feet or less?" he asked.

"Close," I answered. "I triaged him, started an IV, and got lab work."

"How long were you that close?"

"About ten minutes. I saw him again today and we talked in the hallway for a bit. What the heck is going on, doc?"

"You need a test. Go to the decon room and wait there. Don't leave until the ED doc comes to talk to you," he said.

I waited for a while in the decontamination room. I wondered what in the world was happening. A nurse came in with a long Q-tip and proceeded to shove it up my nostril almost all the way to my brain! That was horrible! After I regained my composure, she went for the other side! Oh, heck no! Even after 45 minutes, I felt like that stick was still up my nose.

Finally, after four long hours, the physician came in. "Hey Grover, I know you must be wondering what this is all about. Let me explain. When the patient was here initially, we did not have a test for this new virus the media is talking about. Now we do. And he is positive."

As he continued to describe more details, I didn't hear him. My mind was ringing with the words virus and positive.

Once he left the room, I called my wife at home in Colorado to tell her what was happening. Sandra is a physician and has followed the reports on this new coronavirus infection. The updated CDC guidelines recommended that healthcare workers should be wearing masks at all times in hospitals to protect against this virus. Nobody here wore masks at all, except those patients who were coughing and got a surgical mask in triage.

I hoped my test wouldn't be positive for this, because I might end up as a patient in the hospital. What would having this virus be like? How would my wife handle this so far away? I was here to treat patients, not to become one. Yet, I was sitting on a gurney in the decon room.

Finally, I was told my test was negative. Due to my exposure to that sick patient with this disease, the hospital sent me to quarantine for fourteen days, as per the CDC protocol. On my way out, I told the health care staff nearby the information Sandra texted about the new CDC recommendations. One doc got up from his chair and immediately put on a surgical mask.

It was a dark and dreary evening, matching the thoughts going through my head. This thing could turn out so badly if I got this infection. Sandra is in Denver and I'm so far away. I could die from this and she would never see me again.

We don't know anything about this virus yet. I didn't think there were any cases here. We don't know how to treat it. We don't know how to prevent getting it. I was thankful my coronavirus test came back negative, but how reliable was this test anyway?

I told Sandra I was a little upset I had to be locked up—not just in a condo but confined to one room for fourteen days. Growing up as a Black southern country boy, I'm used to wide open spaces. It felt like I was going to an actual prison. As I drove to the condo, I noticed there weren't as many cars on the highway as usual at this time of night. Maybe people were starting to feel the tip of the iceberg after hearing CDC updates in the news and staying home just in case.

Once I arrived, I did what I always do after work; wash all the germs down the drain in the shower. I told the couple who owned the condo where I rented a room that I would be in quarantine for two weeks. They speak very little English, and I speak very little Spanish, so I broke out the translator app on my phone. It worked beautifully. They understood the extent of my imprisonment and said they would do anything to make me more comfortable.

March 5, 2020

I really didn't think it was in New Jersey yet. I thought the virus would take more time to come all the way here, if it ever would. Since I had nothing else to do, I read and learned a lot about this new disease. The first confirmed case in the US was detected in the state of Washington on January 21. The first death in the US was February 29. Cases were escalating rapidly on the west coast. Many casualties were residents of nursing homes. It made sense it would spread fast in close quarters like that. The president seemed like the spokesperson for the daily White House briefings and kept assuring us everything was fine and controlled.

The Korean man was our first case here. At this hospital. Now I read that on March 3 in New York, there were two confirmed cases. The day after he first showed up at our door. And these two cases were not related to travel from China, indicating it was spreading fast in the community. It had been circulating beyond our shores since December. But we were assured it was contained in the US. Who knows where else this has been percolating?

In Italy reports said the virus was detected in Rome on January 31 when two Chinese tourists tested positive. I found it interesting how the country immediately suspended all flights to and from China. The third case occurred a week later when an Italian man moved back home from China. Clusters were identified in Lombardy and Veneto by February 21. Their first death was on February 22.

The virus was also detected in Spain on January 31 when a German tourist tested positive in the Canary Islands. Community spread began by mid-February and by early March, all fifty provinces had confirmed cases. The entire country was put immediately on lockdown.

When I saw that sad news, I knew tourism and travel would be bad for spreading this disease. It's like the flu. It starts in one part of the world and sweeps over the planet. This part of being a global community I'd like to do without. Until now, the USA had been mostly spared. Not anymore.

March 7, 2020

Since I'm a travel nurse, I came to New Jersey from my home in Colorado. I had worked here many times last year and liked it. When I first arrived for this specific assignment, I got a taxi in New York and the driver was a nice middle aged Dominican man. We talked for a while since we were stuck in rush hour traffic.

I asked, "Where do you live in New York?"

"The Bronx. It's a cool place to be," he replied.

"Even though I'm working in New Jersey, I'd love to live in New York just for the experience. It's so close."

"I have an extra room available, if you need a place to stay."

Now he caught my interest. No need to look for a longer-term rental. And if his wife was as nice as him, they'd be great housemates. I asked, "How much?"

When he told me, I was amazed and said, "Hell yeah! I would love to rent the room."

It was a third of the price I was paying in a hotel. I checked to see exactly how far it was from the hospital, so I could gauge my time and distance to work with rush hour considerations. In New York, traffic gets really messy. This location was perfect, just twenty minutes away. I could only think about how it would be living the life of a New Yorker. Initially, I thought this would be a great spot to be a tourist on my days off. I didn't plan on being sequestered immediately for two weeks.

It's only been a few days and I've been hearing nurses expressing frustration and fatigue at the huge volume of patients coming in. These patients were not just ordinary sick, but really sick. This infection was nothing like anyone had ever seen before. Many patients couldn't breathe and got put on ventilators right away. In just a few days, the ICU was almost full. Everyone continued to push on through their exhaustion and work to the best of their ability. Then they'd go home for a few hours, just to return to be engulfed the next day. I hope the reading I was doing, along with Sandra's research, will help when I get back into what is quickly becoming a mosh pit of coronavirus disease.

I started a group chat with the nurses at the hospital to share about how this new virus was from the coronavirus family. It has been around for thousands of years. This specific virus was coined last month as COVID-19: "CO" for corona, "VI" for virus, "D" for disease, "19" for 2019, representing when it first was discovered in China. The dramatic information we got from the Chinese government described thousands of patients getting sick and quickly deteriorating. The staggering volume of patients was only overshadowed by the severity of this infection. Lots of people were getting very sick, very quickly. Obviously, this thing was highly contagious and devastating. There were new articles and reports several times daily on how this was unfolding. It was almost too fast to keep up with all the information.

If I was at work, I would be running around caring for the sick. I wouldn't be able to read up on the new updates and guidelines. This was already getting out of control, and it had only just begun. I told my wife that COVID-19 would probably go down in history as notorious as the Black Plague. She agreed.

Sandra is in charge of a group of doctors serving fifty rural hospitals across the US. As part of her job, she was now spending many hours each day researching the evolving CDC recommendations. The information she sent to me was mostly regarding the importance of personal protective equipment (PPE).

I passed the information along to our doctors and nurses here in New Jersey. Basically, we were getting ready for an avalanche, though in reality, the rapid slide had already started. As health care workers, we needed to be protected. Who would care for patients if we all got sick? Staff members started wearing the recommended equipment from the moment they walked in the door until after they left work. Unfortunately, many had already been exposed and were either sick or asymptomatic and in quarantine. The hospital was still scrambling, but now everyone seemed to be on the same page, with the same level of heightened awareness and caution.

I spent my time in lockdown alone in the condo. I cooked my own food, besides what the landlord's wife would leave at my door. I would get three phone calls a day from the occupational medicine nurses or representatives checking on me to ensure I was inside and not breaking quarantine. They had me check my temperature each day and asked if I had any symptoms.

I was happy I brought my weights from home, so I was able to work out in my room. That kept me busy for about two hours a day. I spent the rest of my time researching more about this situation that was enveloping the world.

March 8, 2020

New York was now the epicenter of the virus in the US. I started thinking that I needed to get my Black ass right back home and out of this city before they closed it down. I made friends with quite a few nurses at the hospital who checked up on me to see how I was feeling. I was luckier than the other staff who worked a few days ago. Four were in the hospital, and two were in the ICU on ventilators.

March 9, 2020

I have been asked many times how I am still married with a schedule like mine. Having a strong relationship to start with is important. Having common goals such as paying off bills or saving for a special vacation is also important. We keep it solid by communicating every day about everything. Nothing is left for secrets—well, except presents and good surprises.

One of the things we came up with during my travels was movie date night. Since there are so many streaming platforms available with access to thousands of films, we can always find something that neither one of us has seen. We start by picking a genre or specific actor, then look at those trailers. We make a selection, queue it up, and get on the phone. After we hit play at the same exact time, we hang up, and text with reactions to the scenes like, "Oh my god! I can't believe he said that!" or "Oh sh#@. She is kicking his ass!" It feels like she is right there with me. Afterwards, we get back on the phone to say goodnight. Communication is the key to not getting sideways with your mate. Beside every good man stands a better woman—I don't want to mess that up. After researching information on this unbelievable virus for hours and hours, it's nice to have date night to connect with my love even though we are long distance.

March 10, 2020

The news was saying that Italy's COVID deaths were surging. By the beginning of March, the virus spread to every region. Despite their overwhelming suffering, I have been mesmerized by what they did as a country. In an effort to boost morale, Italians in lockdown sang opera and patriotic songs on their balconies to one another to strengthen their sense of national pride. It brought tears to my eyes and it seemed like they were singing to me right here in the Bronx while I'm in quarantine watching them on my computer. Their country is synchronized with music, a beautiful and heartbreaking sight at the same time.

Since their schools were locked down, the kids in the neighborhood left notes to their neighbors saying hang in there or stay strong. China responded in solidarity with Italy by posting videos saying *jiayou,* meaning add oil or keep fighting.

Italy had a coordinated medical response by publishing intensive care triage protocols and medical ethics recommendations to the entire country. What will we do in America? Will it get that bad here? I am not sensing a unified effort so far. Our leaders still say they have a handle on things. Not to worry. But do they really? It's the opposite of other information I read on the internet.

I passed my time exercising and thinking and waiting and wishing I could be with my wife. She was diagnosed with stage four breast cancer in May 2019. It was not the genetic kind. Just bad luck, I suppose. It has been a grueling time for her. She had to take a toxic four-drug chemotherapy regimen that took four long months. Sandra lost so much weight during that time because she couldn't eat or drink hardly anything. She said it felt like she had razor blades in her throat and stomach. As a physician, she knows how much food and liquid she needs to consume daily and was unable to get close to that amount. She was definitely malnourished and dehydrated.

Thankfully, I was home on the day my love needed me most. I was mowing the lawn and saw her outside on the deck enjoying the sunshine in the mild Colorado summer weather. The sun was warm, but sometimes could get intense. I saw her go inside. Our daughter was home, and I heard her yelling for me to come quickly. Oh god! My wife was on the floor in the hallway, pale with her eyes closed. She looked dead, but I could see she was breathing. Elise is a paramedic and just like her mom, calm in the face of an emergency. By the time I got inside, Elise had already assessed the situation and knew what was wrong. Sandra started to come around and was quickly able to answer questions appropriately. She was embarrassed because she pooped on herself when she passed out. There was no way she would let me or our daughter help clean her up. What a fighter! We took her to the hospital to get checked out. She received IV fluids and was sent home. It was amazing how hydration perked her up. She was back to bossing us around in no time flat.

When she finished all that chemotherapy, she needed to do radiation that burned her skin pretty badly. After that, she had numerous surgeries because of infections. Then IV antibiotics and more surgeries. When she was diagnosed, I had already committed to a hospital in New Jersey for intermittent short assignments. The hospital was accommodating with our situation and let me work all my shifts for the week back-to-back, so I was able to fly home twice a month. It was expensive, but being able to see her every ten to fourteen days made my traveling gig tolerable.

Our kids are grown responsible adults. They helped take care of her when I was away, so I didn't worry too much. Luckily, she survived the chemo, radiation, and surgeries. Now we are waiting for May to get her scans again. The doctors are cautiously optimistic that she might be one of those that live twenty years or more with maintenance treatments. She is strong and will beat this, I just know it. She has to.

March 11, 2020

I've been in lockdown for about a week now. I heard nurses in the hospital started dropping like flies. Almost half the nursing staff and residents at this teaching facility were in quarantine. The culture of hospitals quickly changed here as well as around the rest of the country. Emergency rooms told people not to come to the ED if they exhibited mild symptoms. It was best to stay home. Only come if your symptoms became worse.

This ER went from seeing 500 patients a day to only about forty. But those few were really sick. Our ICU was overwhelmed, just like all the other ICUs in the state. There was nowhere to send the overflow.

March 12, 2020

Yesterday in an Oval Office address, the President said that for the majority of Americans, the risk of contracting coronavirus was very low. That was not our reality. Many medical professionals were in the hospital as patients. More were in quarantine, like me. This was already out of the "very low risk" category.

I saw online the WHO just announced a global pandemic and was "deeply concerned by the alarming levels of spread and severity" and was worried about "alarming levels of inaction." There were no widespread guidelines in this country for containment.

Because things got derailed so fast here in New York, the governor started a curfew. Anyone caught out on the streets would be fined and punished by the law. This was an effort to keep people from mingling and spreading this awful disease.

Since I shared the kitchen and bathroom with my housemates, I wiped down everything every time I went in there. My landlords were gone most of the time, so I was able to go into those rooms when needed. They worked day and night driving a cab and grocery shopping for money. Like many immigrants, they worked hard, lived modestly, and sent most of their earnings back home to support their families.

Looking back, I would have followed a different sanitizing protocol. Thankfully, I didn't accidentally expose my landlords. It would have hurt them financially to be quarantined for half a month. And it would have been on my conscience if I passed the disease to them.

There has always been a need for travel nurses across the country to temporarily assist in hospitals that are short staffed. This year, we have been unable to keep up with the demand. And now here I was stuck in one room for two weeks, unable to help because I was exposed when we were not prepared. We in the medical field knew the virus could potentially spread to the USA. There was no way to understand what that would exactly entail. Now that reality is here, it is beyond anything anyone imagined.

Soon it's going to get so bad we will run out of space in the hospitals. There will be a shortage of PPE, testing supplies, and, of course, healthcare workers very, very soon. Medical professionals will get burnt out quickly and if they all get sick… there is no back-up plan.

March 13, 2020

We read about other pandemics in history classes like the Spanish flu in 1918 that killed 50-100 million people around the world. In 1957 there was an Asian flu where 1.5 to 2 million died. Then the Hong Kong flu in 1968 when one million people didn't survive. The viruses that caused these outbreaks have been identified as H1N1, H2N2, and H3N2 respectively. The H and N represent certain proteins on the virus with names that are like Greek to me (Latin to be more accurate). H1N1 was the first. The next mutation was H2N2 because both proteins were changed. The third mutation was H3N2 because just the H protein changed that time. And we were finding out COVID was 100 times more lethal than H1N1.

We seemed to have gotten a handle on influenza, but now here was this coronavirus and our planet has completely changed in three short months. Our current generation has never had to live through a natural disaster like the infections that decimated the world throughout the last century. Maybe that is why some people are sucked into the conspiracy theory, thinking the pandemic is manmade and intentional. This is all Mother Nature. It's frightening to see twenty-first century scientists and global leaders scrambling to find the best way to handle this. But that is science. It doesn't find the answer in seconds. It takes time, and initially mistakes could be made that can be corrected with trial and error.

March 14, 2020

The crisis across the world was still growing. Spain imposed a national lockdown today. I wished I could get back to the trenches to help my fellow nurses overwhelmed by this pandemic (although that's not yet the official classification used by US officials). I felt like I was in a straitjacket in quarantine while others are out there suffering. I couldn't do my part. Another side of me was still worried I might show symptoms and turn positive. There were so many unknowns, it was hard to stay calm sometimes. But physically, I felt fine.

March 15, 2020

I only have three more days, then I am free. I never thought I would ever see those sci-fi movies come to life and yet here I am. This raging plague, as well as being stuck in a room away from my family, made me question about being in nursing. What got me into this field in the first place?

As a young Black boy growing up in Lucedale, Mississippi, I fully expected I would end up working at the shipyards like all the grown men in my family. These men were big and strong, just like what I wanted to be when I grew up. They provided for their families by putting a roof over their heads and food on their tables. Everybody knew they would never get rich working at the shipyards, but eventually they could get to be supervisors. It was one of the very few long-term jobs available in the area, if you could put up with the work and the risks.

At eighteen, I joined the ship fitting apprenticeship program, even though I knew details of the risky job. If you had to wear steel-toed boots and a hard hat, there must be some degree of danger involved. In this place, someone got injured every day. Sometimes it was a minor thing, but other times it was not. I heard about people who slipped off the icy deck, hitting the pavement a hundred feet below. They never survived that.

A lot of people lost their fingers, but it didn't seem to bother them much because they knew their value. Pinky fingers were worth $2,500, other fingers were $5,000 cash. I went to the infirmary one day after a minor injury and a man came in with his thumb cut clean off. He was actually smiling because he knew he was going to get $10,000—a third of his yearly salary. Despite the good money, I would hope that shipyard workers would do all they could to keep their bodies intact. You eventually run out of accessory parts.

My brother also worked there. He told me folks regularly passed out while welding in small, cramped spaces during the hot summer months. It happened to him and many of his co-workers numerous times. Even though I heard the stories of people getting hurt and dying on the job, I was young and thought it would never happen to me. I was happy making $9.60 an hour, more than what most other young folks were making. I fully intended on staying for the long run.

One cold winter morning, I was cutting into an aluminum bulkhead using a "suicide saw." The saw hit the bulkhead at a weird angle, bumped high in the air, and slammed down on my knee. I couldn't look! This was how guys lost their leg on the job. Screw the money, I wanted to keep my body in one piece! I dropped the saw on the ground and opened one eye to see. Everything was still all connected, but there was so much bleeding everywhere. My supervisor immediately took me to the infirmary. The doc didn't seem phased at all when I was carried into the room dripping red. He tended to the big gaping wound on my right knee and twenty long stiches later, I went home on crutches.

As soon as I walked in my house on my own attached two legs, I kissed the wall, happy to be alive. I wanted to live my life with all my fingers and both of my thumbs. I wanted to keep both arms and both legs. I knew this job was not for me. No way! I never went back. Even to this day when I go home to Mississippi, my sweet sister, Charla, always says, "Hey Nicky. You remember the time you came home from the shipyard and kissed the wall? Boy, you were so happy to not be workin' at that shipyard anymore." I love her for reminding me to always be grateful.

As a typical teenager, I wanted to be just like my older cousins. It was a rough crowd, yet every young boy looked up to them because they were cool and always had money. They smoked dope and sold drugs. There were lots of all-night parties with dancing and drinking and plenty of girls. Since I was family, they let me hang out with them, even though I was the youngest. I could have money, cars, girls; whatever I wanted. All I needed to do was exactly what they did. That life sure was easy, but I didn't realize it was just as dangerous as the shipyards, maybe even more so.

There was always drama with my cousins. It seemed we were inevitably starting something with somebody. There was a new guy in the group who looked pretty darn rough, like what you would see in a modern gangster movie. They told me to get in the car to go with them to some small town in Mississippi. Usually I just followed along, but this particular day, I had something to do. I don't remember what it was, but it must have been important enough for them to let me off the hook. I heard a few days later they ended up robbing a guy and shot him in the head. The stranger got caught and went to prison. That could have been me! I could have been the one who ended up in prison or even shot in the head, if I had been there.

We went almost every weekend to my uncle's nightclub. One night, things quickly got out of hand. My cousin, Drake, ended up getting in a fight with a rival gang over his ex-girlfriend. People pulled out guns and randomly started shooting, bullets flying everywhere. We ran trying to get away like every other person in the joint. I bumped into my brother-in-law's cousin, who just got out of prison. He put a gun to my head and said, "Muthafucka, I don't know you, and I don't care to know you. I'll blow your fuckin' brains out right here, nigga."

You hear people describe times when their life flashes in front of their eyes. Well, it happened just like that. It was like an old projector reel playing random scenes in a silent, slow-motion picture; my childhood, funny practical jokes my brothers did, my momma cooking in the kitchen. I knew I was a dead man standing and closed my eyes. Drake showed up just in time. He yelled, "Hey nigga, that's my cousin! Let him go!"

As gun shots continued to go off, I ran out the door with my life. We jumped in the car and drove away. Drake still shot at the guys in front of us. I had no idea who he was shooting at or why. I felt right then I could end up as a statistic—dead by the age of twenty. I had to get out before it was too late.

Black men in the South die young and this was one reason why. Others in this same situation left and got an education. Why couldn't I do the same? My two older brothers went to college and were not in the gang scene. They had families and didn't get shot at every weekend. But first, I had to figure out what career would be right for me. Engineering? That was interesting, but required too much math. Business? Too vague and seemed boring. My pop was a boom truck operator, which was one of the higher paying and safest jobs on the yard. Since I quit, there was no chance of that for me. He also was a Methodist preacher man. That career was definitely not for me, either.

In contemplating this dilemma, I remembered my momma always made sure we all went to the doctor when we were sick and to the dentist for regular check-ups. I grew up without fear of those doctors and wanted to be like them, even though those professionals were White men. They both seemed to like their jobs and I knew they made enough to have a comfortable life.

My dentist had money and pretty girls working in the office. Boy, was he smart! He was not getting shot at or running from the police every weekend. Maybe being a dentist wasn't exactly what I was looking for, but I started to realize that something in healthcare felt right to me. When I looked at all the possible healthcare fields, nursing was the fastest way to get what I wanted. In just a couple of years I could be working in a career that would be both financially rewarding and professionally satisfying.

After I got my degree and worked a couple of months in nursing, I joined the Air Force to help pay for the rest of my education. During my six years there, I finished my bachelor's degree as a Registered Nurse and rose from an enlisted airman to the rank of First Lieutenant. Working in the medical corps in the military helped me develop my ability to adjust quickly to situations. It was the same as working in a regular hospital, except we had to be ready to go to the front line, if needed. I am certain that experience will help me to adapt well during this emerging COVID eruption.

March 16, 2020

I kept tabs on the tall Korean man and heard he would be leaving the hospital soon. He was the first patient I knew with this awful disease. But he was young and strong. I was glad to hear he would recover. I know young folks will probably be more resilient to this disease, but it wouldn't be every one of them. Many of various ages, in good or bad health, would die in this crisis.

I also thought I was invincible until that accident at the shipyards and when I got a gun put to my head. That same foolish thinking will make kids not pay attention to the seriousness of what's happening now. They will bring the virus home to their families and kill the ones with weak immune systems, including their elders.

March 17, 2020

The last state holdout for coronavirus cases was West Virginia. Now all fifty states have been affected in an astonishing short time. It was unbelievable how quickly this disease had spread. It seemed like some alien mutant was taking over our planet. In reality, it was a natural virus that traveled with people. Now that air and cruise travel are commonplace, it spread faster than any virus was able to spread before. People travel all the time and go all over the world in a day or two. Look at history. Soldiers during WWI traveling on ships and trains helped bring the Spanish Flu to uninfected areas of the world in 1918. Otherwise, that devastating virus would have died out long before it spread.

Americans over the entire country were suffering and needed support from our leadership. Laws were passed to provide money to American families making $75,000 or less per year. The first wave of checks will go out by April 15 and our tax deadline will be delayed. This will definitely be a boost to the economy.

What wasn't a boost to the economy was that the CDC recommended a worldwide shut down on cruise travel. But think about a petri dish of a ship in the middle of the ocean with crew and passengers from all over the world in close, tiny quarters. There are hundreds of ships with thousands of people on each. Where are they going? ALL OVER THE WORLD! A little stop here, a short stop there, and there you go—coronavirus propagation explosion.

March 18, 2020

More countries closed their borders trying to contain the virus. I wonder if we were acting fast enough as a country here to avoid total disaster. But the border of my room was open. My quarantine was finally over! Now it was time for a different kind of war than I experienced in my past. Under normal circumstances, this hospital in New Jersey was one of the busiest locations I had ever worked in with their 100-bed ER. My co-workers told me that I would not believe it until I saw it.

The sudden dramatic change was staggering. This hospital had 775 beds and we had over 1000 patients admitted—all were COVID-positive. Even though people were asked to stay at home for minor things, the emergency department was busting at the seams. Every hospital has a disaster preparedness master plan, but we were definitely not prepared for this. The hospital environment was a frantic mass of disorganized moments of chaos. There was a shortage of PPE, a shortage of ventilators, a shortage of rooms, a shortage of workers in every department, but no shortage of patients.

Now without fail, all hospital staff wore what was recommended by the CDC. This included all PPE—gown, gloves, goggles, and even a head covering to keep coronavirus droplets out of our hair. Some people were using face shields, but those tended to fog up quickly, and we couldn't see what we were doing. Finally, everyone wore masks. Not just surgical masks, but N95s. We should have been doing this weeks ago. Now we had the best chance to be protected.

There was a test to make certain the N95s actually fit our faces to keep the virus out. I put on a mask. The person testing me sprayed a scent near my face. I could smell it, which meant it didn't make a proper seal. I tried another style of mask which did not fit either. To be adequately protected, I had to wear a PAPR (Powered Air Purifying Respirator) while I was in the hospital. Since all the patients had COVID, I had to wear this contraption the entire twelve to sixteen hours per day. The PAPR is a hood with a face shield connected to an air purifying machine. It looks kind of scary, like something you would see in a film about a dangerous viral global outbreak. But that was exactly just what was happening in real life now.

The ICU rooms were filled with sedated patients on breathing machines. Other patient care areas, like the recovery room people go to after having surgery, were converted to additional units for Intensive Care. Usually, this hospital had forty-eight ICU beds and now there were eighty ICU patients on ventilators.

Since the ER was turned into a big ICU, a triage tent was put up in the parking lot. Patients were seen there and either sent home to quarantine or admitted to the hospital for treatment. The ER was always full to overflowing, with additional patients on machines in hallways. Other hospitals in the area were in the same predicament, so we couldn't transfer patients anywhere. The waiting room was full of sick patients yet to be seen with no place to put them, and new patients kept coming.

The hospital closed the OB and Oncology wards to convert them to COVID units. How would patients needing cancer and obstetric treatments be seen? I felt so hopeless, like being lost in the middle of the ocean without a floating device. Several times a day, I had to take a deep breath and shake off overwhelming sensations of sadness and helplessness that crept over me. It was hard, yet I was able to maintain the focus needed to try to keep as many people alive as possible.

March 19, 2020

In this hospital so far, I had only worked in the ED and had not yet personally seen the ICUs. Today, I helped transport a few patients up to those critical wards. It was a sight unlike any other. All the nurses and doctors were wearing hazmat suits, similar to what I saw when I served in the Air Force Trauma Corps. Some patients were in special beds that could invert. Most of the intubated patients were turned prone as a last-ditch effort to improve their oxygenation and save their lives.

Under normal conditions, hazmat suits are never worn in the ICU and here was a unit full of healthcare workers looking like people in space. Nor was it normal to see a ward where most of the patients were on their stomachs with tubes and IV lines coming out of just about everywhere. These patients ranged from young to old. I sympathized for everyone, but especially the young ones who might not make it. The loss of their future hurts my heart. It was quiet and somber with the exception of the rhythmic humming of the vents breathing in and out of each patient keeping them alive. There was very little conversation as those on the care team wore muffling face shields and the majority of patients were totally sedated and paralyzed. I have been a nurse for twenty-three years and it was the first time I ever saw anything like this.

March 20, 2020

California issued a stay-at-home order. It was bizarre to think of an entire state full of people being quarantined. Who knew when they would be able to open again? The governor of New York started the curfew here about a week ago, but I was seeing folks not abiding by this at all. As I drove back to the condo in the Bronx, I passed by parks with people walking their dogs and throwing frisbees. At a basketball court there were twenty guys hanging out waiting to play a pick-up game.

This was madness. People were in denial. I heard some folks saying they thought this was a hoax or that the government was trying to kill Black people and other minorities. They really said this to me. There were even some healthcare workers who thought this thing was not real. I was unsure where those guys worked if they didn't acknowledge what was happening in hospitals, because they couldn't be experiencing what I did.

March 21, 2020

On my rare day off, the couple I stayed with asked if I wanted to help them with their shopping. Since it was an essential service, it was a good way to get out of the house. There was a sudden spike in the need for shoppers since the governor announced a stay-at-home order yesterday. Now everyone wanted home deliveries. We drove to a nearby grocery store and they pulled out their phones. They showed me an app where there was a list of food items to buy for a specific person. It was actually really fun running around like a scavenger hunt game trying to find the exact item in the right size or flavor or color. When everything was found, we checked out, then delivered the items to the customer's door.

This couple made a whole lot of money in one day. It wasn't difficult and I enjoyed it.

We were driving all around upstate New York delivering food. It reminded me of home back in Colorado with rolling hills, a lot of trees, and beautiful green meadows. The drive was quiet and peaceful and serene. It was a dramatic difference from the overcrowded big city with millions of folks crammed in a few square miles. I was sure crowds of people living on top of one another could contribute to why this COVID surge was rising so fast here.

I'm sure people were grateful for the deliveries, but they never came to the door until after we left. At one house a person in a plastic suit from head to toe with plastic booties, along with a hood, goggles, and gloves, came out and wiped down every item before taking anything inside. I could understand this degree of caution. There was so much unknown. There was also so much conflicting information.

There were others who represented the polar opposite viewpoint by believing this outbreak was fake and related to political agendas. Some say it is nothing more than a bad cold. Half of the people in the community do not want to wear masks and the other half do not plan on leaving their homes for months. This pandemic will definitely get worse before it gets better if we don't get unified in our approach to slow the spread of this contagious disease. People need to get on board wearing masks, washing or sanitizing hands, and keeping socially distant. And now, before it is too late!

March 22, 2020

It was easy to see that the nurses, residents, respiratory therapists, and other techs were all burnt out. There was too much to be done. One thing in particular on our to-do list for patients who are intubated was to provide mouth care every hour or more often, if they needed it. These patients had tons and tons of secretions, like I had never seen before. If staff neglected to do mouth care, the patients were put at increased risk to catch additional infections just by being admitted in a hospital. We call these nosocomial infections. These could possibly be prevented if we had more time. We tried to do the best we could and it was never enough anymore.

We have to put in Foley catheters to drain their urine, nasogastric or orogastric tubes to remove excess fluids built up in the stomach. Our kidneys are probably one of the most important organs in the body. We have to keep an accurate count on how much urine a patient produces. Those kidneys are very sensitive and when they fail, other bad things start to happen that cause the patient to spiral downhill.

Rectal bags are commonly used because many patients have constantly running liquid stools. The feces drains down the tube and collects similar to urine in a Foley bag. We push this soft pliable tube past the rectal sphincter and instill about 30 milliliters of saline in the balloon tip, so it won't dislodge. These are just a few of the things we have hanging from all the patient's orifices. Unfortunately, we have to make plenty more holes in order to insert medications or administer treatments to assist with the patient's survival.

When we do CPR on patients, all the organs in the body will be affected in one way or another, even the skin. It is an organ which can tell us a lot about a patient's condition. If the skin is healthy and pink, it tells us there is adequate circulation. If the skin is dusky, grey, or mottled, blood flow is a problem. If blood flow is inadequate, every organ will suffer and start to malfunction—the kidneys, the liver, the heart, the brain. Pushing on the chest is a way to squeeze the blood out of the heart to continue circulating to the rest of the body while trying to save the patient's life.

This brutal practice of CPR has been known to save millions of lives. And I cringe when I feel ribs cracking from a seventy-year-old grandmother during chest compressions, knowing that scattered rib bones could cause a pneumothorax. And it's not just one broken rib. I have cracked three to four ribs doing good CPR technique, especially in the elderly or chronically ill.

These coronavirus patients have gone through a lot and are deconditioned from fighting so hard. They are given life sustaining medications and if we stop any of these IV drips they will crash and burn. Many do not make it.

March 23, 2020

One COVID treatment is the "proning" of patients. Simply put, this is turning a patient on their stomach. There are beds that rotate a safely secured patient so that they are under the bed and facing the floor. Because these beds are expensive, there are so few of them. Most of our patients need this technique done manually. It's important to watch and make sure that all those tubes and IV lines do not get kinked. We arrange the lines in the bed next to their body with the patient's arms down at their side. Then, we place a sheet on top of them covering the patient from head to toe. Next, we wrap them up like a burrito and pull the bottom sheet as we turn the patient on their side with their back to the bed rail. After making sure the breathing tube is securely in place, we flip the patient on their stomach, turning their head either to the right or left. This is only half of the process.

The next step is to angle the bed to have the patient's head up higher than their legs, so they will not vomit. Then we have to position their extremities using the "swimmers pose." On the side they are facing, that arm is down at their side. This is important because if the patient wakes up, they could possibly reach their breathing tube and pull it out if that arm was raised, which is a bad idea. The other arm is up by the back of the head, like a swimmer. The legs are also positioned, one up with the knee bent and the other leg straight down. It only works if the bent leg is on the same side as the lowered arm. I had to lay in a bed on my stomach in this position to really understand how to make it comfortable for my patients. Every hour, we need to switch arm and leg positions, as well as direction of the heads of our COVID patients. Five to six pillows are placed under their torsos and extremities to prevent bed sores.

Why would we spend so much time and energy to turn them over like this? COVID secretions tend to pool in the back of the lungs due to gravity. Those secretions are thick and get stuck closing off large areas of the lungs. The proning position helps spread those secretions around and not let them accumulate in the back, so the lungs can possibly function to oxygenate the blood.

We all have seen hospital shows where the patient becomes unconscious and is dying. The nurse calls a "code blue" overhead and everyone runs in and starts pushing on the dying person's chest. Normally, there are a handful of codes in a large busy hospital per day. COVID has changed this to where there may be twenty or thirty codes every single day in a busy hospital like this. With the use of the proning technique, I saw an immediate reduction in code blues. Some patients eventually were able to get off the ventilators and leave the ICU. Proning definitely helps the life expectancy of a patient in the ICU with COVID.

Driving back every day to my room in New York was now eerie. There were no cars on the highway at night. No people were out and about. There were news and military helicopters flying low over the city. It was strange to see 45th and Madison Avenue completely empty of pedestrians and I was the only car on the road. It really felt like an apocalypse, like in the movie *I Am Legend* with Will Smith when there was no one left in the city. It felt like the world could be ending. But I am far from done. I still have a lot of living left to do.

March 24, 2020

I was honored when Fastaff Travel Nursing Agency asked me to write an article for their national newsletter. It's a great company for me to work for because they have a large variety of positions available in hospitals in several states. I can go just about anywhere.

It was a good thing to share my experiences and hopefully prepare fellow nurses who were getting ready to jump into this COVID catastrophe with us. I described the proning beds and how strange it was to see them in the ICU, although I knew it was potentially saving lives. In my article, I shared how these were patients of various ages. Initially it was reported that the elderly or those with multiple medical co-morbidities were the ones most at risk. While that was certainly true, some of these intubated in the ICU were younger patients between the ages of twenty to fifty. This disease seemed to not be sparing anyone.

Jackie, my recruiter who always has my back, told me how much they appreciated me being able to work in many hospitals across the country, each one with unique situations and challenges. Hospitals consider a nurse to be valuable if they are flexible and can work wherever there is a hole in the schedule. Initially I could be scheduled for an ICU shift, but I could step in if the hospital needed me in another area. I can work in the ER, ICU, Medical floor, Surgical floor, Rehab unit, or in Pre and Post Op.

Several times, I was asked to be in charge of the unit where I worked. Once I filled in as House Supervisor, overseeing the entire hospital. Since travel nurses are transient by nature, we are rarely appointed to these leadership positions. I have worked in so many hospitals that I have practically seen it all and feel comfortable in a management position if the situation calls for it. I want to work as much as possible to distract myself from being far from my family. I'll do overtime shifts if someone calls in sick. I'm happy to work seven days a week. I will go in early and stay late—whatever the hospital needs.

March 25, 2020

Today was the last day of my assignment in New Jersey. I was happy to go home to Colorado. The governor of New York said on the news they could be closing the bridges to isolate the city. This was insane! How would I be able to get home? I couldn't stay here any longer or I might be stuck. Last night I packed up my car. Right after my shift I headed west directly from the hospital.

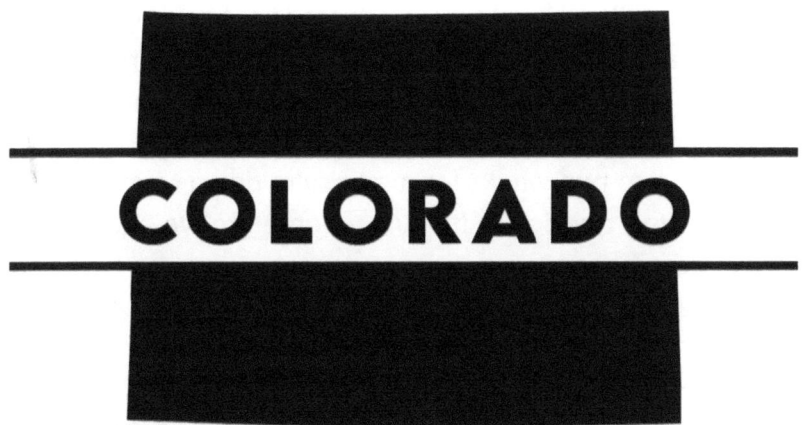

March 27, 2020

On the two-day drive back home, I wondered if I would be able to truly relax. I already wanted to turn around to continue to help those COVID patients struggling to survive and healthcare workers struggling with the overload. But having a break with my wife will help me keep my sanity.

I tried to decompress by listening to good music and chatting with Sandra. I don't realize how stressed and tense I am after a long shift out of town. But Sandra knows. Every time I come home from an assignment, she tells me how I seem to be all pumped up on adrenaline. My voice is loud, and I speak unusually fast. My movements are brisk, and I walk quicker than normal. Usually, she is the one that is dragging me behind her whenever we go anywhere. She says it takes one to two weeks for me to calm down to my regular normal. I don't notice it. It's just a home groove and a work groove difference for me.

Getting outside and doing physical activities also helps me relax. To make everything better, the weather now was typical Colorado–perfect. The days were in the 60-70s and dry with sunshine every day. It was nice to see snow still on the ground from huge recent storms. It was Denver's snowiest March in four years! It snowed last weekend and dumped about twenty inches of heavy, wet snow which still covered the grassy areas.

I was worried about it piling up in the driveway when I was away. Due to a recent surgery, Sandra was on a ten-pound lifting restriction for another two months. Our son, Logan, lives close by. He and his wife Kaitlyn along with our daughter, Elise, came over regularly to make sure the driveway was cleared and that Sandra had everything she needed. In my heart I knew she had good help, so I was worrying for no good reason.

We were coming up on the one-year anniversary of my wife's initial diagnosis. We prayed her scans would come back clear. Waiting and not knowing was the hardest part of this ordeal for me. That treatment of hers was rough. If all is good, we celebrate. If there is still active cancer, we change treatment, and keep going. I was holding my breath and tried to put myself in her shoes. But I'm not the one with the cancer. I cannot fathom what she must be thinking and feeling, knowing there is a possibility this could turn out really badly.

Everyone asks why don't I stay home and work closer to her. Coronavirus was killing people, but cancer patients with decreased immunity were especially vulnerable. Sandra would be more at risk if I worked close to home seeing COVID patients and returned to her every day. It was better to leave for a month or two, then come home for a month or so. This would keep her safer, with less virus exposure, until we get a vaccine.

March 28, 2020

We walk our dogs to the soccer fields near our home almost every day when the weather is warm, to give us some much needed exercise. Today, our Belgian Malinois, Sasha, stayed on leash until we got to the park. She always performs fetch like an Olympic sport. She trembled with anticipation until she was free and we launched the ball. Sasha almost reached it before it hit the ground. When she brought the ball back, I swear she was smiling. If it was up to her, we would spend twelve hours of nonstop play. Belle, our American Bulldog rescue, is never interested in wasting her energy chasing a toy over and over again. She only wants to get her belly scratched and to be with us.

When I was home last December, the weather had warmed up, and I didn't see the frosted meadows like usual. I missed that white Christmas. The snow on the ground today made me feel nostalgic and brought back memories. Sandra finished her chemo last September, had her bilateral mastectomy at the beginning of October, and was in the middle of daily radiation treatments in December. Stage four cancer of any type tends to force everyone involved to reevaluate priorities. I realized I was in danger of losing my love and immediately any squabble became minor. Being with my baby as much as possible became most important. Above all, I want us to be happy. I tell my wife many times a day how she's always right, if only to make her happy—I gladly do it.

At Christmastime the kids came home with their spouses, filling every bedroom in the house. We had agreed beforehand to make presents from scratch. It was great to see how everyone rose to the artistic challenge. Our son, Jacob has a small forge in his shed and made elegant heart-shaped metal ornaments with red ribbons to hang on our tree. Our younger son Logan made an intricate bird house with six rooms and painted it to look just like our home. Our daughter Elise and both daughters-in-law, Hallie and Kaitlyn, made soft colorful crocheted things like hats, scarves, mittens, and socks. Here in Denver, you can't have enough of those cozy winter accessories. Homemade gifts are fun, thoughtful, and made with love. Each time we use the gifts, we think of the people who made them.

March 29, 2020

Every morning, Sandra and I make delicious lattes from our espresso machine. It makes the best coffee. Sandra would know. Her family is from Brazil and she tells me coffee runs through her veins which makes her an expert on this topic. As we enjoy the morning sun, we scan the news articles of the day. At the top of the list we noticed the CDC COVID Tracker. The numbers were climbing daily on an alarming steep trajectory.

Emails started coming in with open positions across the country. I know I need to get back out there soon, but I just got home. I estimate it will take at least three weeks to recuperate and recharge my mental batteries before jumping into the raging coronavirus river again. Without any reliable treatment or a vaccine, I feel completely vulnerable, because I am. This virus is so contagious and I am exposed to a high viral load for twelve to sixteen long hours when I am at work. My co-workers and I are the ones touching the sick while caring for them. Some patients require constant help and each of us have more patients a day than we can safely handle. It's entirely exasperating. There's so much I need to do for my patients, but there are not enough hours in the day to get it all done.

There have been some news reports about hydroxychloroquine (HC) and azithromycin used together to maybe help reduce symptoms in patients with coronavirus infections. As a physician, Sandra has used HC to treat rheumatoid arthritis and couldn't imagine how it would work for this disease. This week, one of the doctors in her group got COVID and had to quarantine in California. She called my wife.

"I'm so sick with fever and body aches. What can I take besides acetaminophen?" she asked.

Sandra answered, "You know there is nothing proven yet to help. If you can't stay hydrated because you are throwing up or have diarrhea, then you have to go back to the hospital and be a patient."

"What about HC? Have you heard much about that? And taking it with azithro?" the doc asked.

"There is no reliable data yet. You know this. There just hasn't been enough time to do a proper double-blind study," Sandra answered.

"Would you take it if you were sick? Be honest, would you?"

"I cannot tell you what to do. We are all guessing at this point. I know the FDA cleared it for experimental use, but it is not tested. We don't know the potential side effects or if it will even work. I don't know if I would try it," Sandra explained.

The doc decided to take it along with the antibiotic. She ended up having side effects of heart palpitations and shortness of breath. Her trial with an n = 1 did not work. It still took four weeks for her to get over the worst part of her symptoms and another two months to get halfway to normal. She put herself in potential danger by taking an experimental medication. A relative handful of patients cannot compare with looking at 50,000 cases. Trying any unproven treatment has risks. The FDA ultimately rescinded their provisional approval for HC due to serious side effects and lack of enough evidence that it works.

March 31, 2020

	COVID CASES		COVID DEATHS	
JAN	Global 12,308	US 1	Global 265	US 0
FEB	Global 86,471	US 60	Global 2,978	US 0
MAR	Global 889,005	US 149,378	Global 45,236	US 5,210

April 3, 2020

The focus in the media has been our economy and how most states issued stay-at-home orders. With only essential businesses remaining open, millions of Americans were immediately out of work. We were quickly becoming a real-life colossal apocalypse with empty streets, businesses closed, and bare grocery store shelves. Many people were saying it's the beginning of the end of the world. Science says otherwise. It is another pandemic like many in history. The other pandemics were devastating and yet resolved. This one will, too.

    I could understand shortages of meats, rice, bread, and canned foods, even bottled water. But toilet paper? There was no bathroom tissue in the whole entire state! Where are people finding space to store all the Charmin? In a few more weeks, I might have to sneak in my neighbor's house to look for their hidden stash. Someone told me there are two different factories that make toilet paper, one for commercial use and one for residential. Since everyone has been staying home and using their personal toilets, rather than at work and public places, residential toilet paper factories couldn't meet the sudden increased demand. Maybe bidet sprayers will become popular here like in most countries in the rest of the world.

April 12, 2020

In a few weeks, I will be going again, but I am not sure where. Every morning, Sandra and I look at job postings for ER or ICU. There are hundreds of shifts now that coronavirus has hit the scene. I know this meant a lot of Americans were dying. It's hard to see this suffering exploding everywhere. Where can I make the most difference?

I needed to figure out which state would be best and make my decision soon. It takes time to complete all the required documents and "competencies" or tests to prove how much I know. Each hospital has their own versions, but it's the same information. If I go to ten different hospitals in a year, I take ten different exams about EKG reading or calculating the rate of an IV medication. Each place will also require another drug test. I have done so many in the last year, the lab must be curious as to why I am there so often.

April 15, 2020

A news report showed how unemployment had risen to an all-time high. In one month, the percentage of people out of work in this country rose from 10.3% to 14.7%. Two and a half million jobs were lost. It had never increased like that in thirty days' time since the 1940s. The "real" unemployment was higher than that because statistics didn't take into account Americans who were under-employed. For example, if a restaurant manager is laid off in response to a stay-at-home order, he might find a job as a delivery driver. He is still making money, but not the same amount that he did before. That "real" unemployment was estimated to be close to 23%. These numbers crushed those of the post WWII era. Have we really been thrown in a massive recession in the short span of four months? Is our economic way of life destined to collapse?

I read the Coronavirus Crash that began on February 20 was a major, sudden drop in the stock market that affected the entire world. This signaled the official start of the COVID-19 recession. An immediate response by the banking industry in major countries around the globe was to cease the decline by easing banking regulations. The Bank of Taiwan announced a $6 billion credit line program to stimulate small business growth. The Bank of South Korea announced a $12 billion funding operation for the South Korean banking system. The South African Reserve Bank announced relaxed regulations, making R300 billion in credit available. The Bank of Israel announced easing restrictions to stimulate lending and economic growth.

Here in the US, we also helped boost the global economy. The Federal Reserve Bank stepped in to mitigate economic long-term damage by lending $2.3 trillion to households, small business owners, state and local governments, and financial markets. The lending interest rate was near-zero with the promise that it would stay that way until labor market conditions improve. Experts praised how this global effort turned the tide away from economic disaster—the life buoy needed to help us ride out this storm.

April 22, 2020

New York was getting hit hard, with well over 30,000 people sick and 2,000 deaths so far. The city finally mandated masks because maskless people riding subways, trains, and buses were a critical factor in the virus spread. Everyone must know by now that being in close proximity to others was the best way to catch this infection. Or do they? There are over 20 million people in NYC/Jersey City crammed in twenty square miles. It is no wonder that it is the epicenter for the pandemic in the US.

When I looked at the assignments available today, I saw a position pop up in New York. This is it. It looked like the hardest hit area was the Bronx, where I stayed before. Whenever I take on a specific job, I give myself 100% to the hospital. It makes for a better assignment when I don't expect anything like real down time. I just bust my ass to get through until I get to see my wife again.

In my few days off I would be able to live like a New Yorker. Despite the stigma of NYC being this busy rat race empire, I still wanted a taste of what all the talk was about. When I stayed in the Bronx when working in New Jersey, I fell in love with the Big Apple. I even toyed with the idea of getting a place in Manhattan, but Sandra would hate living in any big metropolis.

April 23, 2020

Yesterday I saw the White House briefing with President Trump and members of the coronavirus task force. Bill Bryan, the Undersecretary for Science and Technology at the Department of Homeland Security shared that there were ongoing studies that showed increases in humidity and ultraviolet rays, along with bleach and other disinfectants help kill the virus in the air and on non-porous surfaces. President Trump tried to discuss this further and suggested to Secretary Bryan,

> "we hit the body with a tremendous, whether it's ultraviolet or just a very powerful light... And you're gonna test that. And then I see disinfectant, where it knocks it out in a minute—one minute—and is there a way we can do something like that by injection inside, or almost a cleaning... So that you're going to have to use medical doctors with, but it sounds interesting to me.... Maybe you can and maybe you can't, I'm not a doctor."

Today Trump said those comments were sarcastic. The President of the United States has a great influence over many people who will do what he suggests. Like a month ago a couple tried to self-medicate with fish food that contained chloroquine phosphate. The wife said they ate it because Trump discussed the potential benefits in his briefings, and they were scared to catch COVID. The husband died and the wife was in critical condition for a long time. This isn't the same as the pharmaceutical medicine hydroxychloroquine used to treat malaria, which was being studied to see if it could be effective against coronavirus. I hope more people do not take it upon themselves to experiment, no matter what they hear.

April 25, 2020

I had a lump in my throat today. I had to leave Sandra again. At the same time, I had to admit there was a part of me that was ramping up to get back to the action. The long rides in the car to my assignments kept me safer from COVID than flying in an airplane. Besides, I enjoyed having time to think and I liked having my own car to drive around in my temporary home. I was heading back to the COVID war and that mood drew me back to my days in the military. In New York, there wouldn't be any sitting around.

There wasn't much time to sit around when I was in the Middle East either. I arrived in Oman in the winter of 2003 and found the medical clinic was being run out of a trailer. The first order of business was to build a field hospital as quickly as possible. We put up a dental clinic, emergency room, medical ward, surgical suite, and ICU from the ground up in only one week. The time spent there was pretty routine—mostly seeing less sick or lower acuity patients in the hospital, rather than seeing a lot of wartime action.

I loved my job as an officer in the Medic Unit because I had several different responsibilities. I was designated as Infection Control Officer in charge of policies and procedures. It was a little boring since it included a lot of paperwork. I was also chosen to oversee the Honor Guard that posted the colors every morning and evening. Taking care of the flag gave me a renewed respect for my country and the symbol that represents my freedom.

I met a lot of airmen and made decent spending money doing a side gig of cutting hair. The base barbershop charged around $15 per haircut for just getting clippers, buzzing the guy's head and cleaning up the edges. I didn't understand why they charged so much and why each one took so long. I went to barber school years ago and never lost my skills. I had a line of guys waiting for me every day after work and all through the weekends. Those guys tipped me and I saved plenty of spending money for my fun time when I got leave.

Sandra calls often after dark as I drive on these trips. She knows I have a hard time staying awake when the sun goes down. It was late and I saw a motel up ahead. Since I ate as I drove tonight, I just wanted a shower and a pillow.

April 26, 2020

I hit the road again early this morning. After a couple of hours, I stopped for breakfast. I sure missed my baby's cooking already. Then I got back on the highway to return to the COVID front lines. Driving for long hours in the car was never fun. I was missing my daily training. My body needed movement! My mind started reminiscing again about when I was in the Middle East.

Guys were missing their sweethearts, like I was right now. Others missed the adrenaline and wanted to get back to the front. We were stuck on this base and couldn't go anywhere for fun. I wanted to help morale and immediately the answer was clear. Martial arts has always been a passion in my life and part of my routine. The guys saw how I worked out and did my training every day. They asked me how I got into it. My older brother, who I respect and admire, introduced me to martial arts when I was a young boy. That moment truly changed the path of my life. It helped with discipline and developed awareness of dangerous situations. Because of my enthusiasm, I quickly excelled in the sport. I rose to a fourth-degree black belt level in the Taekwondo organization.

As an officer with a black belt, I thought it would help lift the spirits of the troops if we started a martial arts school. The base commanders gave me authorization and I got to work. I contacted ATA (American Taekwondo Association) Grand Master Ho Lee to get permission to open a martial arts academy under his umbrella. I needed more black belts to help me teach the troops, but that would take years. In this unique situation, however, I was allowed to give soldiers credit for previous martial arts experience in styles like Brazilian Capoeira, Kempo Karate, Shotokan, Krav Maga, and Isshin-Ryu. In a short time, I had ten black belts trained and ready to go. It was an honor to have all the necessary permissions by ATA Headquarters to proceed. They even waived the $30,000 franchise fee.

Our academy grew to over four hundred students in just one month! We had class four times per week in the evenings after work. I had to stand on a podium and use a bull horn, so they could hear all the instructions. Our school was so successful that I was told we were on the cover of ATA magazine, along with a big feature article describing TRAB (Thumrait Air Base) ATA Black Belt Academy. The troops loved having this physical and mental outlet. It helped keep their focus on something positive, rather than getting depressed or finding creative ways to wreak havoc.

I was jolted out of my daydream by road construction eliminating lanes and traffic cones everywhere. My car has larger than normal tires, so my speedometer isn't completely accurate. Cars were passing me on a regular basis, so I knew I was not speeding. A cop pulled me over. He came to the window and asked for my license and registration. As I passed him my documents, I showed him my nurse badge and explained I was on my way to New York to work. Politely I asked why he stopped me.

He said, "You were going one mile under the speed limit." The cop told me to get out of the car and go sit in the cruiser so "we could talk."

I knew to tread lightly because the look of distain on his face was clear to me. He was in a position of power and could pretty much do what he wanted. He asked, "Do you have any weapons or drugs in the car?"

"Of course not," I answered.

He asked, "If I call for the canine unit, would they find anything?"

"Definitely not, sir."

I must be a drug dealer being a Black man driving a bad ass BMW with Colorado plates in Chicago. Why else would he pull me over for driving one mile below the speed limit? He asked to search my car and opened all my suitcases. That man rifled through everything, leaving a big mess. The last bag had a lock on it. Once he saw the lock, he figured the pounds of drugs he hadn't found yet must be in there. With a suspicious look, he ordered me to unlock that bag.

I explained it wasn't actually locked and asked him to simply unzip the bag. "My scrubs are the only thing in there, sir."

After not finding anything, he handed me my papers, and said I could go. Before I left, this White cop asked, "By the way, how in the world can YOU afford an expensive car like THIS?"

If I were White, would he really have asked me that? If I were White driving this car, would he have stopped me for obeying all the traffic laws? As I drove away, I had the feeling of being totally violated. If he were injured or sick and came in my ED, I would do everything I could to save his life regardless of his race. I am not about retaliation for the historic slavery of African people or for what some narrow-minded individuals may think. My skin color has not prevented my success. I just want to live a long loving and peaceful life and be judged by the value of my actions instead of how I look.

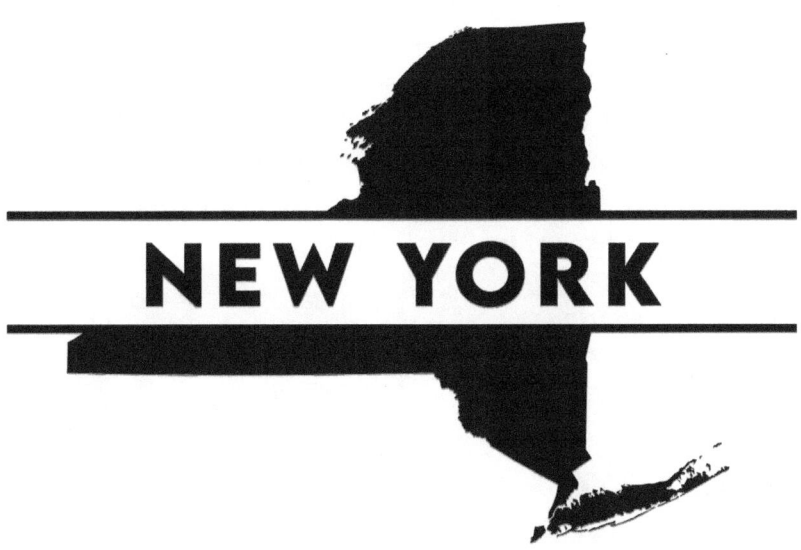

April 26, 2020

The streets were still almost empty when I arrived in New York. It was obvious things were bad here in this desolate metropolis.

My assignment is in a large hospital in the Bronx. The Roosevelt Hotel is free to healthcare workers and not too far from my hospital. The hotel is beautiful with nice marble floors and huge chandeliers. Even though it is aged with a slight musty smell, it still maintained its elegance. The rooms are big enough for me to bring my spin bike and weights. When I made my reservation, they explained how the gyms were all closed with the state's shut-down order. They were designated as unessential, but working out is always essential to me. It helps me blow off steam from an overwhelming COVID day and keeps me levelheaded.

April 29, 2020

Usually, a hospital spends a week orienting new nurses to the workflow, computer system, hospital policies, and protocols. Mine lasted two days, and we hit the floor running. Every day before I went to work, I stood in a long line at the staffing office to get our work assignments. After that, I stood in another line waiting to get my N95 mask I needed to use for the entire day. Masks were in high demand and in short supply. The hospital was tightly regulating who got them and how many. There was talk around the hospital that our supplies would last only a few days. News reports were saying the entire country was running out of everything—masks, gowns, and gloves. How would we as healthcare workers be protected from this infection if we ran out of PPE? It would be a hazardous work environment if we didn't have the equipment to be safe as we performed our jobs. It seemed there should be a reasonable solution here. Why couldn't the government appeal to companies to restructure factories to make more masks? There could be a tax break for this. It would be a win-win-win situation; the hospital would be able to buy more PPE for employees, the manufacturer would get paid, and the patients would get treated. We needed to figure this out quickly. This is just the beginning. We cannot run out of supplies—and so soon!

Walking through the hospital, I asked about the photos of people on almost every wall—mothers, fathers, and entire families. I was told they were memorial walls of all the staff and their families who died from COVID-19 so far. Hundreds of people from this hospital alone have already died in just a couple of months from this horrible disease—doctors, nurses, therapists, and some of their loved ones. What is going to happen throughout this year!?!

April 30, 2020

I had been working in the ED the last few days. Today they switched me to the ICU. As I walked to the unit after getting my N95, I looked outside. There were some semi-trailers in the parking lot. "What are those trailers for?" I asked a co-worker.

She responded, "You'll find out soon enough."

Later on during my shift, a patient on the unit coded and died. I was asked to help take the body to the morgue. We went down the service elevator, down the back hallway, and out the doors into the parking lot. Those semi-trailers were huge coolers for the corpses. There were over two thousand dead bodies out there, all on individual gurneys in overlapping rows. The hospital morgue had filled to capacity long ago.

This is now real-life scary in the US of A! What is happening here?! I had seen similar things in the third-world, but not in my first-world country. I could be one of these statistics, dying from a COVID exposure away from home, and end up in one of those trailers. I have to focus and do the job I signed up to do. I have to help those sick patients as best as possible, but also, I have to stay protected.

	COVID CASES		COVID DEATHS	
JAN	Global 12,308	US 1	Global 265	US 0
FEB	Global 86,471	US 60	Global 2,978	US 0
MAR	Global 889,005	US 149,378	Global 45,236	US 5,210
APR	Global 3,482,232	US 1,086,625	Global 238,993	US 62,955

May 2, 2020

I knew I was here for a specific reason—a mission. The general response to a pandemic is something we in healthcare had talked about and prepared for since I can remember. Nobody really believed it would get to this level of a crisis. My first day here in the Bronx was just last Monday. My life was on the line as well as those lives of all my patients. I felt like I had been thrown right into the deep end not knowing how to swim in these waters. In the other hospital I wore a PAPR machine, due to the masks not sealing well on my face, but in this hospital it was not available. I was putting myself at a greater risk, but what could I do? I wore an N95 and a surgical mask together. Would that be enough?

As nurses, we all know how to put on a gown and gloves. Now we were being shown a very detailed COVID way to wear them. The putting on procedure is called "donning" and taking off is called "doffing." Supposedly, this specific and detailed way to put on and take off PPE was the best to reduce our chances of contaminating ourselves and avoid spreading coronavirus to our scrubs and skin.

DONNING PPE: Wipe hands with sanitizer, pull on a pair of gloves, put on the gown. Then place face mask and either a shield, or goggles. Put on another set of gloves to cover the top of the gown sleeve cuffs.

DOFFING PPE: Grab the middle of the gown about stomach level and hold it away from your body. Start rolling up the gown into a tight ball, letting it come loose from your neck and waist. Next, take off the first set of gloves inside out and stuff the rolled-up gown inside them and throw that away. Wipe the face shield off with sanitizer, then remove. Take off the second set of gloves and throw away.

Just the donning and doffing was exhausting, much less doing actual nursing care. Can you imagine having three ICU patients, each one requiring going in and out of the room several times an hour, 24 hours per day? I did the math in my head and saw immediately this PPE process was not sustainable. There were over 6,000 hospitals in the US and if they all used PPE like this, we would run out in less than a month. Factories couldn't possibly make enough for this explosion. What would we do for protection then? Can you imagine the healthcare worker shortage if we all caught this disease because we simply didn't have enough PPE?

May 3, 2020

I had to fill my off days with other activities besides riding my spin bike and lifting weights, so I decided to start a new hobby. Who would ever think that a tough Black man like me, veteran, fourth degree black belt, trauma nurse would love grocery shopping for people? I was surprised to find it so addicting! Every day when I was off work, I scanned shopping orders for the ones I liked best. There are certain stores that have items easier to find. I don't understand why some stores put canned tomatoes in a different aisle than the canned veggies or the lemon juice in a different aisle than the other juices. Larger orders were great since I could stay in one store for a longer time. But sometimes the short little ones that I could do quickly were fun too. It's amazing I made a lot of extra money each week working six or seven hours on my days off. This could be a great solution for people who lost their jobs during this crisis.

May 4, 2020

As I entered the ICU to go to work today, it was frantic. Everyone was running around, and things seemed to be noisier, crowded, and in disarray. Beeping IV pumps were outside the rooms now, which was not the norm. Usually, IV poles are plugged in the wall behind the patient's bed inside their rooms. The new protocol was to use extension tubing to keep pumps in the hallways, so nurses could reduce the number of times they had to enter a COVID environment. Changing a bag of fluid or medication could be managed from outside the rooms. It seemed like things were chaotic. In reality, our days became more efficient. These COVID-19 patients were extremely contagious and labor intensive, so the less time we spent in their direct space, the less chance we had of getting COVID. It is so needed and necessary to think outside the box in many aspects with this crisis.

COVID patients needed care at least once every hour which required putting on a gown, gloves, goggles or face shields, and hair coverings. Sometimes we were in a patient's room for three to four hours—giving medications and trying to stabilize them in addition to performing specific routines for basic hygiene. There was the mouth care protocol to perform every hour on patients who are intubated. We also had to bathe them, clean up after bowel movements, and reposition them every two hours, so they didn't get bed sores.

After finishing with one patient, those PPEs were taken off, and new PPEs were put on to go into the next room. The process began all over again. This, of course, doesn't take into account when patients decompensate. There were so many emergencies every single day that took us away from the routine care. If a code blue was called, we stopped what we were doing, took off the PPE, ran to the other room, put on new PPE, and entered to help. Just to put all this in perspective, we now have about fifteen code blues in a twelve-hour period when we used to have fifteen in a month. It was no wonder when we got to the end of the day there were things we didn't get to do. I always hated leaving tasks for night shift, but I couldn't stay there forever without sleep. Instead of *c'est la vie*, the saying should now be *c'est la COVID*.

There wasn't enough time in the day to finish required tasks, much less taking the time to document everything in the patient's chart. No wonder the unit seemed like a live pinball machine. Nurses bouncing around from place to place to place, trying to care for patients, dealing with beeping IV pumps and alarming monitors, charting in the computer about everything that has been done with each patient, answering phone calls from doctors and families, among a myriad of other duties. We joined forces in teams where each nurse got a buddy to help with tasks hoping to work faster. It was the only way to hopefully complete the job in twelve hours, then leave to be able to sleep, just to return the next day to do it all again.

May 8, 2020

By now, burnout was starting to affect the nurses. Everyone seemed depressed and overworked. They were crying more often—in locker rooms, with patients' families on the phone, and in break rooms. Nurses were also yelling at each other. It was beyond obvious that we were all stressed out.

Administration understood the staff was working past their limits on a daily basis for way too long, so they made sure we took our breaks. There was an hour for lunch and another 45 minutes spread out during the day. This time away from the grind helped us rejuvenate to be able to push through to the end of the shift. Someone told me there were an additional 1,500 travel nurses at this one hospital to help with the higher capacity of admissions and the higher acuity of patients. And we could use a lot more. If anyone still thinks this pandemic is a hoax, they should be admitted for delusion.

While I was home, I read about how the USNS Mercy docked in the Port of Los Angeles on March 27 and the USNS Comfort was deployed to New York harbor on March 28. These Navy hospital ships were supposed to provide additional resources for our overwhelmed hospital systems. Theoretically, it appeared like a quick response by the federal government to this outbreak and a much-needed relief valve for the highly impacted coastal states. When they arrived, we were told they intended to only take "clean" or non-COVID patients to make room for us to care for those infected with coronavirus. What the heck?! We didn't have many patients without coronavirus, so how would this be a help to us? Those Navy ships had the capacity to take five hundred patients, of which one hundred could be very sick needing ICU level of care. They really could make a significant impact on our struggling local medical communities, if they would just open up the hatches.

It was astonishing to me that the USNS Mercy treated only seventy-seven patients in six weeks. They will depart Los Angeles on May 15. The USNS Comfort removed half of its one thousand beds, so they could have room to isolate and treat coronavirus patients safely. On April 21, Governor Cuomo told President Trump the ship was no longer needed in New York. While docked in the city, it treated less than two hundred patients.

In early March, the Army was deployed in New York. They are now in my hospital to assist us on the units. They started bringing in meals every day for everyone. This simple gesture of appreciation made me feel excited and upbeat as it got closer to lunchtime. We all smiled trying to guess what would be the food choices of the day. There were a variety of delicious meals with plenty of leftovers that would normally be thrown away. At the end of my shifts, I went down and grabbed those leftovers for the homeless people close to my hotel. Some did not want hand-outs. Once I even got food thrown back in my face. Most, however, were grateful for the gesture.

May 10, 2020

Even though I was available to work every day, the hospital only needed me three to four days per week. Travel nurses usually are paid more than employed nurses at a hospital to compensate for the travel burden and being away from families. Besides offering a higher hourly rate, the hospital pays a living stipend and expenses. In addition to that, the travel agency gets their cut. Usually, a hospital will anticipate how much time a nurse will be needed and will contract for a specific number of hours per week at a certain rate. Generally, hospitals will avoid scheduling that traveler for anything extra. It becomes overtime and paid at time and a half. I am certain this will change as the virus spreads. Hospitals will need every available healthcare worker every single day. And I predict it will happen soon. This will be so expensive for the hospitals, but also for the patients receiving weeks and months of costly treatments. How is this financially viable?

May 12, 2020

In non-COVID times, nurses on a regular hospital floor can reasonably take care of four to six patients per day, depending on how much care they need. For example, a patient who is admitted for a little dehydration or mild pneumonia needing some IV antibiotics and oxygen for a few days is easy. However, a patient who is paralyzed from a stroke will require more attention since they have to be repositioned every two hours, administered all their medications and treatments, get range of motion exercises on their affected extremity, and given their meals. An ICU patient takes even more time with additional numerous medications and therapies, suctioning and respiratory treatments, along with bending and stretching every extremity, and changing their position more frequently, so they don't get bed sores. Usually, the patient-to-nurse ratio in an ICU is 2:1, unless the patient has special circumstances requiring 1:1 attention.

COVID has blown up all those usual ratios. Nurses on the floor are seeing six to eight patients daily and ICU nurses routinely have three at one time. Not only are these COVID patients sicker and need much more attention, there are also a lot more of them. And there are fewer staff members available due to burnout, sickness, or mandatory quarantine due to COVID exposures. There are not enough nurses to go around, or respiratory therapists, or nursing aides, or x-ray techs, or lab techs, or housekeepers, or administrators. And patients keep coming.

May 14, 2020

There was one travel nurse who had been here longer than me. She seemed friendly and always asked how she could help. She offered to reposition patients or flush IVs. She even tried to give medications and hang antibiotics, but I never let her do that. She went above and beyond, but something about her rubbed me the wrong way. One day she made a comment to me saying she needed to relax and go smoke some weed. I definitely needed to keep my distance from her.

Several days later, she was found not breathing in the bathroom with a needle in her arm. She overdosed using medications she diverted from patients. She coded three or four times in the bathroom before the team was able to get her intubated, stabilized, and transferred to the ICU. There were four vials of Dilaudid in her pocket. I don't know what happened to her, but I hope she survived. If she lived, I am sure she would end up losing her nursing license and likely would go to jail. It's so sad to see this happen to a colleague, especially when we need all the trained nurses we can get.

May 15, 2020

Today the Trump administration officially announced Operation Warp Speed. The main objective is to have a vaccine by January. Other countries are working on this as well. In the US this effort was started on March 27 as a public-private partnership to facilitate and accelerate the development, manufacturing, and distribution of a COVID vaccine. Back in March Congress funded a total of $1.8 trillion through the CARES (Coronavirus Aid, Relief, and Economic Security) Act, $10 billion allocated for vaccines. While the proposed timeline is super-fast, it might be possible given that scientists already have decades of knowledge in the basics of this technology already. They apply that knowledge to this particular virus, do studies, and bam—they have a COVID vaccine. The distribution and vaccination of every human in this entire world, or enough to achieve herd immunity, is something that makes my head spin. I'll trust the experts on that.

On top of the high demands of patient care, there were daily conflicts regarding minor issues such as a cart being placed in the wrong location or a patient not being transferred out in a timely manner. Maybe a room wasn't cleaned fast enough. Petty issues constantly intruded into our day that was already challenging enough. As I heard the constant bickering, the Bobby McFerrin song kept swimming around in my head, "Don't Worry, Be Happy."

May 17, 2020

Today I received report from the nurse going off duty. The patient was a 43-year-old female who walked into the ER yesterday talking and able to communicate like she would any other day. She was admitted to the regular floor for shortness of breath, body aches, fever, weakness, fatigue, and a few other complaints along with COVID.

The charge nurse from night shift told me that the patient got put on BiPAP in the night. This is a Bilevel Positive Airway Pressure machine, which helps push air into and out of the lungs. She continued to worsen and was intubated just before shift change at 0700. I walked to the door of her room, which was strange that it was closed. When the ICU is full, the critical patients will overflow to the Medical Surgical unit. Those units are for people not as sick, so there are none of the fancy monitors feeding vital patient information to the nurse's station. You would never have a patient on a ventilator in one of those rooms with the door closed because you have to watch them constantly. I opened the door and I looked onto an endless sea of trash. This is a common thing in a busy trauma room or when a patient is coding. You do not have time to throw things away properly in the moment. Save the patient first and clean the room later. But this messy room was not cleaned at all. I heard a few codes being called as I walked in, so I was sure the team had another patient to save and left the cleaning to me.

I surveyed the rest of the scene. Her intravenous fluids were empty, as well as all the sedation and pain medication bags. I had to move fast in order to keep this patient from waking up and extubating herself. She needed to be in a room with a monitor. In order to move an intubated patient, every team member has to be ready to help. We need the primary nurse, respiratory therapist, and another person or two, depending on how many IV poles need to go with the patient.

I called RT to help transfer this patient to a room across the hall. It had a monitor, even though it wasn't ICU. Respiratory therapists are under-recognized throughout this disaster. They are the main professionals swimming in this sea of mucus and sputum. I always acknowledge their commitment and dedication to keep patients breathing. As usual, they too were short staffed with a full house of COVID patients requiring respiratory treatments, suctioning, EKGs, ABGs, among many other tasks they had on their plates. It took a while for RT to get to me, but we eventually got the patient moved and settled.

I was finally able to hook her up to a monitor and check her vital signs. Her blood pressure was 60/28—not good. This was not a life-sustaining pressure. Her heart rate was 30, which was also not good. I immediately called a rapid response. It isn't quite a code blue but will silently call in a resuscitation team to stabilize a crashing patient. The team usually consists of a doctor, charge nurse, primary nurse, respiratory therapist, pharmacist, and a couple other staff members who are all certified to administer ACLS (Advanced Cardiac Life Support) algorithms to try to save a life.

We were instructed to start chest compressions per ACLS protocol and give epinephrine. This amazing drug brought her back for a brief five minutes. She was put on several medications to help assist her blood pressure and heart rate. Then she crashed again. This all started around 0800 and lasted until 1400 in the afternoon. I could not leave her bedside for one minute until after 1500 hours.

I had to insert a Foley catheter to keep close track of her urine and an orogastric tube to lavage and decompress her stomach from air and gastric secretions. The ED doctor placed a central line, so I could have enough IVs for all the medications she needed. Putting in these catheters, tubes, and IV lines are standard and common practice for most critical patients. In the middle of this, we had to make certain we were protected against the misting and floating air droplets of the corona bug. Finally we got her assigned to an available room in the regular ICU. However, in order to get into that room, I knew a COVID patient either got better or more likely, was sent to the morgue.

Since every patient was corona positive, we had to wait for housekeeping to decontaminate the space. The last hospital in New Jersey required rooms to be closed off for an hour before being safe for environmental services to enter. Just like all other departments, housekeeping was short on staff, too. We had to wait for her ICU bed for three hours before it was finally cleaned and ready. Then we transferred this patient to an appropriate ICU room with the typical modern technology.

Unfortunately, a few days later, her fingers and toes started to turn black, her kidneys started failing, and she puffed up like a balloon. Her legs were weeping serous fluid on the bed sheets. We put ice packs under her arms, under her breasts and pannus, and under her legs because her temperature rose to over 104°. The patient died after three days of treatment.

Her husband was out of town. The last time she spoke to him was on her way to the hospital in the beginning of all this nightmare. When he came to pick up her personal effects, he asked for her cell phone. It must have gotten lost during the move or somewhere in all that trash and commotion. This sometimes can happen, and we were very sorry. She had special photos and videos on that phone, and they were forever gone.

I especially noticed throughout my ICU experience with this virus the majority of patients who have greater problems are obese, with diabetes, high blood pressure, renal disease, heart disease, or have chronic respiratory issues. There are also unexplained anomalies in patients who are younger and in good health; they too can become extremely sick and die.

The primary reasons patients are getting admitted to the hospital for COVID is because they did not follow guidelines of social distancing or did not wear a mask. There are also some who might have been trying to do what was right, yet became infected by a family member, friend, or maybe someone they barely knew. They could have picked it up inadvertently by not paying close attention to protocol when opening a door in a public place, then using their phone or scratching their nose without cleaning their hands first.

Patients who did not make it out of the hospital alive cannot go back in time to fix what happened. I can't speak for all nurses, doctors, or health care professionals, but for me, the feeling of fear goes through my mind every day when I am on shift. When I put on my PPE, I start to feel anxious. My heartbeat quickens when I enter the doorway of really sick ICU patients. I can feel death overtaking the entire room. If I didn't have a mask, I am certain I would be able to smell it. It is the most eerie perception, knowing death is eminent. It encapsulates my body and is in the air like I can almost touch it. I know I am doing what I can to protect myself every day so hopefully, I won't catch this awful virus.

May 20, 2020

Today was my wedding anniversary. I sent flowers to Sandra to arrive this morning. Instead of being home with my wonderful wife, I was working and assigned to the Burn ICU. This is the hardest of the ICUs because these patients are really suffering beyond what any patient should endure. My patient was one of the worst off I have ever seen in my entire career. His body was charred with fourth degree burns over 40% of his body surface from smoking while changing out a propane tank in his camper. Not only was he burned beyond recognition, he also had COVID-19. We kept him on IV sedation continuously, but the meds sometimes ran out.

If I was occupied with another COVID patient, I couldn't always hear the IV pumps beeping in another room. If there was even one minute delay in his sedatives, he was wide awake and in pain. In addition to closely watching the timing of all his meds, his dressing changes alone took over two hours every day. As with other COVID patients, he had copious secretions and required frequent suctioning. I could have spent my entire twelve-hour shift in just this one room and still not finish everything I needed to do for him. But there were two other coronavirus patients needing my attention.

Most COVID patients in the ICU were on many drips requiring close monitoring to ensure there was no gap in infusing the meds. They were on Fentanyl for pain, Propofol for sedation, a paralytic drug to help them not fight the ventilator that was helping them breathe, blood pressure drugs to help keep their pressure up when it was trying to bottom out, multiple antibiotics, antiviral medications such as remdesivir, steroids, and blood thinners in addition to their regular home meds.

We've been using an experimental treatment of plasma donated by people that have had a COVID-19 infection and fully recovered. The idea was they likely had antibodies that could be helpful in treating COVID patients in the hospital, especially critical ICU cases. I felt a sigh of relief because now there was an additional way to treat patients other than remdesivir. The drawback was that we ran out of blood products almost immediately. There is a public plea for plasma donations from previous COVID patients. I hope everyone who can donate will help.

This job really requires a special type of person with all grit and heart. Nurses, doctors, therapists, and various ancillary healthcare workers are special in their dedication to take care of patients in this dangerous environment. It's like how we worked in a war zone when I was in the military. The triage tent outside the hospital is similar to the temporary medical clinics constructed in Iraq or Afghanistan. It is natural for us to be afraid of this, but fear does not mean a lack of action. And this is a war that will eventually end, too.

Despite the overwhelming numbers of patient deaths within this short time, there are still people in the community refusing to acknowledge the reality of this virus, the sequelae of this pandemic. There are people who don't believe any of this is real, though so many patients are getting extremely sick and dying. Some are even doctors and nurses around this country. Many don't intend to get the vaccine when it is developed.

The only way we are going to win this war against coronavirus is for all of us to work together against this common enemy. We need to do everything we possibly can within our power. Wearing masks and practicing social distancing everywhere we go is vital. Even when we are at home with our extended families, we need to wear masks and stay a safe distance away and clean our hands every time before we touch our faces. Soon enough we can have a huggy sing along, but for the time being, sing it to yourself in the shower. Better yet, do a group webchat and sing there. We all need to socialize and in the safest way to help me be able to spend future anniversaries in person with my wife.

As I left the hospital, Sandra called. I answered with, "Happy Anniversary, baby."

Sandra said, "I've been waiting all afternoon to call you. I have some news."

My heart skipped a beat. It had better be good news, especially after this rough day. "Um, is it good?"

"Well, I got the results back on my scans."

"What are the results? Is it good or bad? Don't leave me hanging, baby," my heart beat faster and my breath quickened.

"Well, I got the CAT scan of my chest and it was clear. But I also got the CAT scan of my liver—and yes, it was also clear."

"So, what? There's no cancer anywhere?!?"

"Nope, no cancer!" she exclaimed.

"Wow, baby! You went from stage four to no sign of cancer, in one year! That's so great! We have to celebrate extra when I get home." I felt like clouds carried me back to my hotel. The rest of my night I could only think about my love and I was so grateful I could be with her longer.

May 26, 2020

All over the news was the murder of George Floyd. He was killed yesterday by the police. It was incredibly senseless. This brought back memories of that cop who pulled me over on the way here. That man could have done something similar to me.

There were worldwide protests against police brutality and racism, and the lack of police accountability for their actions. Floyd's death came after the killing of Breonna Taylor on March 13. I hadn't heard much in the media about Breonna Taylor, which says a lot about what is important in this society. After looking into her death online, I found that Louisville, Kentucky police used unwarranted and exaggerated deadly force, and a black woman died. In February, an unarmed Ahmaud Marquez Arbery was shot and killed by three White neighborhood residents. Have we regressed this far? Or has this been happening all along; one killing here, one killing there, and it doesn't make the news?

As a Black man, this shocked me to my core. Floyd was being arrested for allegedly using counterfeit money. After getting handcuffed, the officers tried to put him in the back of their vehicle, but Floyd fell to the ground saying he felt claustrophobic and couldn't breathe. The officers struggled to put him back in the car, so instead Floyd was placed face down on the ground with an officer's knee on his neck.

Floyd continued to complain about breathing difficulties. Bystanders pleaded for the officer to lift his knee and help him. The knee stayed on his neck. Floyd said he was about to die and even called out for his mother. He eventually stopped speaking. For another two minutes, he lay motionless. Only after they checked for a pulse and found none, was the knee removed.

I have heard people say, "If you don't resist, you won't get hurt." Videos supported the fact that he was not resisting. Why is he dead then?

This incident sparked organized protests. Thousands of people were gathering at the site and placing candles, notes, and flowers. This could be the start of permanent change, like when Rosa Parks refused to give up her seat on the bus. She was far from the first person to refuse to give up her seat, but she was the spark that led to big changes.

May 27, 2020

I have PTSD and night terrors from my time in the military. The ones where I am paralyzed and something is trying to smother me to take my breath. It feels like I will definitely die in my sleep. I can't do anything to wake up, no matter how hard I try. Now we are all living a similar nightmare with hospital beds full of extremely sick patients who can't breathe and can't wake up. And staff running around going out of their minds, not knowing when this will end. Once vaccines are developed there will be a resolution to this madness, but that's a long way off.

Every single human is affected by this crisis in some way. Some have lost social gatherings, others lost their jobs, others their businesses, some lost family members, and there are many who lost their lives. And on top of this global medical crisis, we are suffering with social and political unrest. Why is this all happening? When will this all stop? The best I can do is hunker down and do the most I can for my patients, then go to sleep, and it starts all over again. Same thing but a different day.

May 29, 2020

This virus has been affecting humans for only five or six months. The CDC still doesn't have much information about it or how to treat it effectively. It's no wonder why cases are still rising all around the world. Our hospital was overflowing. Our ICU was full of vented patients and now, we ran out of ventilators. Four entire floors were converted to units dedicated to the care of COVID-19 patients. Other spaces like waiting rooms were converted to patient care areas as well. No one can visit anyway.

We still wore the recommended gear, even in the break rooms. N95 masks were in very limited supply, so the CDC put out guidelines to extend and reuse this necessary piece of equipment. This is not optimal as extended use reduces how effective they are, but we can't run out.

Despite all the agonizing despair, there were several positive developments I saw in the last month. We now have a Rapid COVID-19 test available. This is very important to be able to quickly identify and isolate in just a few minutes those patients who are positive. There are also medications in Phase 3 trials being used for those who are sick in the hospital.

Another great thing is that here, like in New Jersey, there are a few beds that invert, making it easier to prone patients.

Most need to be turned manually here as well. Proning has been used for severe Acute Respiratory Distress Syndrome (ARDS) since the 1970s, but it was rarely done and only in specialized hospitals. In fact, I have never in my entire career seen a prone ICU patient until two months ago. Now it is commonplace and widespread all for COVID.

I saw health care workers rise to the challenge by working above and beyond their usual capabilities. Patients and families showed gratitude and appreciation. Restaurants provided meals to health care workers. It became more commonplace for grocery stores and other businesses to implement social distancing by marking where to stand every six feet in check-out areas and everyone who entered was required to wear a mask.

None of us alive has ever seen a global disaster such as this. We are definitely flying this plane as we are building it. I pray for all of us to keep positive thoughts, and that we match those thoughts with actions in our daily lives to support one another through this tragedy.

May 31, 2020

I saw online that JAMA Ophthalmology reported today that COVID-19 could be transmitted through the eye. I guess we better all be wearing serious eye protection. I wonder what else we will discover about this horrible virus before this is over. Will it affect children differently than adults? Will it affect women differently than men? Only time will tell.

	COVID CASES		COVID DEATHS	
JAN	Global 12,308	US 1	Global 265	US 0
FEB	Global 86,471	US 60	Global 2,978	US 0
MAR	Global 889,005	US 149,378	Global 45,236	US 5,210
APR	Global 3,482,232	US 1,086,625	Global 238,993	US 62,955
MAY	Global 6,515,313	US 1,856,560	Global 382,743	US 108,439

June 1, 2020

The riots in New York made me feel like I was in a third-world country. In fact, my world dramatically changed from my initial contact with the Korean patient in New Jersey back in March. With COVID-19 and demonstrations sweeping the country, what other bizarre things will happen in real life?

I do not remember the street I was on, maybe it was Madison or 2nd Avenue. I was having fun with the scavenger hunt shopping to bring groceries to people who didn't want to go into a packed store. I followed the directions on my navigation to a family located in downtown Manhattan. As I crested a hill and came to an intersection, I heard loud voices and looked up the road.

A huge throng of thousands of people were filling the entire street a few blocks ahead. It reminded me of the walking dead. It looked like thousands of zombies marching towards me at a slow lumbering pace. When I say thousands, I mean tens of thousands of folks, and they were holding signs and were loud.

In New York, you cannot make a right turn on red. Crazy, right? I hesitated at the light for a brief moment, then decided I better just run it and deal with a ticket from the automatic cameras later. Right then, about twenty big black and white vans with NYPD on the sides with running lights and sirens zoomed by. The vans were hauling ass. It shocked me to see the police driving that fast in the city. The speed limit was 20 mph and they had to have been going 50 or more. Police troops on the ground gathered in full gear.

The crowd halted abruptly as someone who suddenly stopped after sprinting to the edge of a cliff and realized there was a dangerous drop a half step ahead. As I waited, I had to come up with a strategy on how fast to make that right turn once the street cleared and the light changed green. As I looked up, it was changing red again. The cops and the sea of people broke my concentration. I missed the light and was stuck. But the mass crossed the street and surrounded my car. I could not turn.

As they screamed shouts of injustices and Black Lives Matter, I saw all different shades of skin, from ebony to caramel to cream standing shoulder to shoulder. Hardly any of them wore masks. They were certainly not socially distanced and looked like lava slowly enveloping everything in its wake. I saw mostly White policemen with some Blacks and Latinos in formation with riot gear, side by side. I held my breath. This could have gone from bad to horrific with just one shot.

Even though I was still surrounded by the mob, I sighed with relief once I realized—wait, I am a Black man. The crowd was on my side. They saw my big mug through my tinted windows and knew I was a brother. Several people smiled and motioned for me to make that right turn which I so needed. It was hard to remember I still had groceries to deliver.

Once I approached the townhouse, I sent a message to the shopper that I arrived. This big burley-looking White man came to the entrance. He made a few comments about what was going down and said he really appreciated what I was doing to help him and his family. This was unusual because most folks waited until I pulled away before coming outside in full MOPP gear to retrieve their goods and products. But this White man came out to intentionally thank this Black man for delivering his food, all while a mob was marching down the street in racial protest a few blocks over.

June 2, 2020

One of my patients today was a woman who only spoke Spanish. The tele-translation support service at this hospital is labor intensive and difficult to use, so most nurses manage as best as they can without it. The patient was obviously irritated when I came on shift. She was shaking her head in refusal of everything I was trying to ask. She even took off her BiPAP and tried to leave the hospital. As soon as she got out of bed, she passed out and I had to call a rapid response. Her O2 sats were 63%. After we stabilized her, I found a Spanish-speaking nurse on another unit and asked her to help me figure out what was going on with this lady. If we could do one thing to make her happy so she would remain safe in the bed wearing her oxygen, what would it be? She started speaking really fast in an animated way to the Spanish speaking nurse, "The food here is so gross! I can't stand it! I'm supposed to eat to stay strong to fight this stupid disease and I can't even put this food in my mouth. All I want to do is throw up when I smell what they bring and put in front of me. I'm done with all this. Completely done!"

Such an easy solution! I called her daughter and asked her to bring Dominican food cooked from home three times a day. This lady's entire attitude changed. She found energy to start participating in her therapies and her condition went in the right direction.

June 5, 2020

The protests were growing around the country and some were turning into riots. There was footage showing when some peaceful protests were ending, violence was started and encouraged by White nationalists. They hid behind signs supporting justice for George Floyd. Were they taking advantage of the unrest to instigate looting and destruction? There were pictures of pallets of bricks conveniently nearby. Who put them there? The peaceful protesters? And get this, a large number of them wear aloha shirts as part of their uniform. I wonder what people in Hawai'i think about that. The group said they are at protests because they hate the police and that takes priority over their White supremacist views. I cannot believe this is actual real life!

Regardless, the spark for permanent change is growing. The four officers involved in the death of George Floyd were arrested. I kept thinking about all these implausible, and yet actual events while I was caring for my patients. I respect the Black Lives Matter movement which was formed out of a grave necessity from social injustice. I am Black. I personally know. And I also researched the data to be certain I don't just have a biased view. Unacceptable police violence can be seen against other minorities at higher percentages than toward White men. Male Latinos and Native Americans have one and a half times those of Whites to die in this type of confrontation. However, confirmed statistics show Black men are about 2.5 times more likely than White men to be killed by police. This disproportion clearly shows what we in the Black community already know—we are targets.

These highly publicized gross examples of minority targeted abuse by law enforcement, are not the only forms of racism in our country. The Asian community is not spared. Elderly Asians are increasingly being attacked at random. Can you imagine going out to get your groceries and someone knocks you down, just because? Chronic systemic racism is more prevalent and rarely reported. In my opinion, it is the root of this abuse we are seeing on the news. I have experienced racism on a daily basis while growing up in the South. My time in the military was a welcome relief because I was less judged by the color of my skin. I live in Colorado and not once have I felt discriminated against in my all-White neighborhood. As a travel nurse, I go to many different hospitals in several states across the country. I have experienced unfair treatment on occasions that would have never happened if I were White and I will not work in certain states as a result. I hope a solution can be found and soon. All of us deserve it, Black and White, and every shade in between.

June 6, 2020

When patients are intubated on a respirator, they need to be on tube feedings for nutrition. This presents a whole host of issues that also absorb much of a nurse's time in a day. The patients need to get finger sticks often to make sure their blood sugars don't go up. The tube feedings usually cause loose stools or diarrhea, so the patient constantly needs to be bathed, and the beds changed. Eventually, a rectal tube is placed to prevent skin sores and breakdown due to stooling. The rectal tube can kink, which will cause a leak and another bed change.

COVID patients on a ventilator need constant suctioning to get copious secretions out of their lungs. Honestly, we can suction every minute of the day and still not get all the mucous secretions out of the tube. If we suction too much, it can cause bleeding in the lungs. If we don't suction enough, the patient has mucus plugging their airways.

Occasionally, we are assigned a CNA (Certified Nurse Assistant) to help us on the unit. The CNA can do finger sticks in most states, empty urine catheter bags, change rectal tube bags, and help bathe and reposition patients. A CNA cannot give medications or do suctioning, but their assistance can free up enough time so we can document in the patients' charts.

June 9, 2020

The medical examiner's findings showed George Floyd was positive for COVID and he had hypertension and heart disease. Also, he had blunt force injuries to his head, face, shoulders, hands, and elbows, and bruising on his wrists consistent with handcuffs. The toxicology report showed evidence of cannabis, fentanyl, and methamphetamines.

Floyd's family ordered a private autopsy and concluded his death was by "homicide caused by asphyxia due to neck and back compression that led to a lack of blood flow to the brain." The body-cam footage showed the true time of neck compression to be nine minutes and thirty seconds. The Fentanyl could have added to the problem, but it did not cause his death.

Floyd had a criminal record. He was arrested nine times, mostly for drug and theft charges. I have heard people say, he was on drugs and the officers couldn't control him. There are enough videos clearly showing otherwise. Even if he was resisting and on drugs, is that a reason to justify him being killed?

This entire story is reminiscent of something that might have happened on a southern plantation over a century and a half ago. Haven't we matured as people as well as a nation since then? What are some people afraid of if minorities are viewed as equals? Would those people be less than who they are now?

June 12, 2020

I am feeling ... overwhelmed is not even close to describing it. I think about our global situation and don't have words. Some people are out of work and bored. Others have too much work. Some people are stuck in their homes. Others are stuck on cruise ships that are not permitted to dock. I heard suicides are up. Humans are social animals. It is tough on all of us. If we have more patience and believe we will get through this, things will be easier. The more people wear masks, clean hands, and social distance, the quicker we will get through this catastrophe. People ignoring safety protocols will bring consequences to us all—especially the weak and us healthcare workers on the front lines.

June 15, 2020

The riots went on for weeks. They would die down, but you would still hear things were getting worse in some areas. I heard stories that vandalism was rampant throughout cities. Innocent people and businesses were affected. The videos and news clips of the clashes between protesters and police were disturbing and unnecessary. I remember seeing a cop push this older White man down and he hit his head on the concrete with a loud crack. He ended up with a brain injury and fractured skull. He is recovering, but this entire situation could have been easily avoided.

You remember the movie *The Green Mile* with Tom Hanks and the big guy Michael Clarke Duncan? I wish I could take everyone's coronavirus away like that huge Black man healed folks. God rest his soul! Maybe we could take away the ills of our social and political unrest, too.

June 17, 2020

Just to complicate matters I read that foreign businesses are flooding the US market with products for COVID. Two Hong Kong-based companies received warning letters from the USFDA and Federal Trade Commission to cease selling unapproved products online in the United States claiming they can diagnose, prevent or reduce symptoms, or even cure COVID.

Then there are the other scams of fake websites selling products that would never be sent in reality. It seems to be happening more often, maybe to prey on the confusion created by the pandemic? Sandra complained that she was getting tons of emails from PayPal, Amazon or Amazoon, and Citibank, among others. They claimed there was a problem with her account and tried to get her to click a link on the email. A big clue was the bad grammar. It's sad that thousands of Americans are falling for these and are losing money.

Also don't forget about the door-to-door con artists selling COVID related items and testing supplies, along with a whole plethora of other goods. I don't know about you, but I wouldn't open my door to anyone I didn't know in a lockdown. I am appalled that in this widespread outbreak, with every country in the world gravely affected, companies and individuals would be this unethical in taking advantage of public fear. Who are we becoming as a society?

June 18, 2020

It is now coming to the end of my assignment in New York. I noticed in the media there was something stirring up in the United States—a conspiracy theory. Every patient I had cared for in the ICU so far were either Hispanic or Black. I had seen very few White patients in this hospital or in New Jersey. There was information all over the internet about this virus affecting more minorities than Caucasians. Was this because of the color of their skin? Or their genetics? Or maybe the fact that minorities were socially and economically disadvantaged living in close quarters and more susceptible to virus spread? Was it that minorities suffered more from diabetes and other underlying health-related conditions, making them more likely to be admitted with severe coronavirus infections? Experts know living and working conditions can affect a person's health. If a subset of the population lives in crowded conditions, they would more likely see a faster spread of a viral disease; like in multigenerational homes seen more in Latino, Asian, and Black communities. Living in densely populated areas certainly makes social distancing a big problem.

Another issue is many minorities work in essential businesses, making them more exposed to the public. This is inherently increasing their risk of contracting the virus. Many minorities also rely on public transportation to get to work. This further increases their potential exposure. Taking all this into account, I guess it is not so surprising we were seeing more minorities admitted to the hospital with COVID-19 infections. I doubt the amount of melanin in their skin has anything to do with it.

June 19, 2020

Juneteenth, Freedom Day, Liberation Day, Jubilee Day, Emancipation Day. This is a holiday celebrating the emancipation of those who had been enslaved in the United States. June 19, 1865 was the day of the announcement by the Union proclaiming freedom from slavery in Texas. Modern celebrations have been with food and music festivals, street fairs, and cookouts. This year, the somber remembrance of Juneteenth was pronounced. Thankfully, the majority of demonstrations that occurred were peaceful, but firm in the resolution that this habit of police abuses would no longer be tolerated by the people. Aren't we in the twenty-first century with the ability to go to space? It is interesting to see how close we still are to the 1860s in this respect.

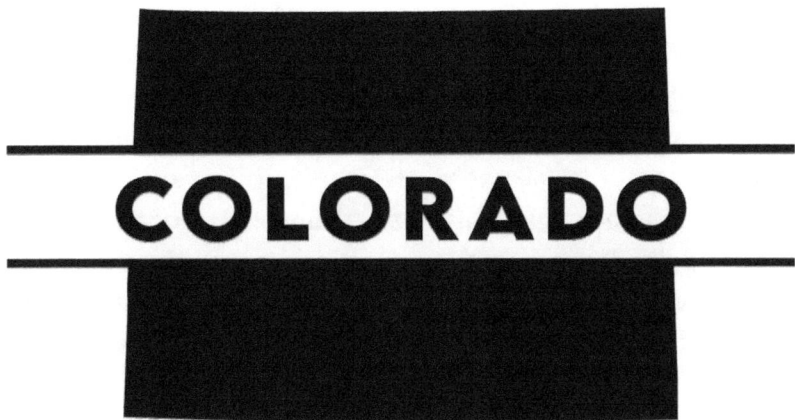

June 22, 2020

I decided to fly from the Big Apple to Denver for a short recoup before I go to my next assignment in Florida. The situation there is dire. Before I go into that unknown, I need to see my beautiful wife and restore. It made more sense to fly than to drive all the way to Colorado and then all the way to Florida. I would spend more time with my love that way. Wearing our N95s, we could enjoy our company in the same room at a distance from each other. Across the room Sandra is better than no Sandra.

Flying has always been a passion of mine. I dreamed of being a pilot, so I went to flight school. Only then did I realize how terrifying it was to think about pummeling to the ground. There was a flight instructor in his 70s who had the most experience out of all them. He started off every class with videos of plane wrecks. This was very unsettling for me. I raised my hand like I was in grade school and asked the question I am sure was on everyone's mind. "Why do you show us these videos of plane crashes every evening before class, sir?"

He replied, "I want to show you future pilots the things not to do when you are in the air with nothing but 20,000 feet of space between you and the ground."

It was most disturbing when they told us flat out the pilots crashing in the videos had twenty to thirty years of experience in the air. I don't know about anyone else in the class, but I was convinced right there and then that my Black ass would take this last exam and be done with pilot school. I just couldn't risk that one chance of being responsible for not making it safely to the ground, for me and my passengers.

I found out that some newer planes are made to autocorrect when they go into a stall. This one safety element has saved many lives because stalling is one of the leading causes of fatal plane accidents. It made me feel more comfortable flying with the big boys as a passenger.

However, with all the insanity that has happened this year, one thing that really made me not want to travel by plane anymore was this dang coronavirus. What went through my mind the entire flight was that the air was recirculated. I held my breath when the guy two seats over had a coughing spell. I felt like I was sitting in a thick pudding with nothing but coronavirus swimming all around me.

OMG... did someone fart?! My damn mask wasn't working right! I turned the little vent knob above my head to allow for the contaminated cabin air to flow downward. Maybe it would blow all the germs to the floor before penetrating my N95 and cloth masks. Once we made it safely, I wanted to kiss the ground. Maybe it wasn't such a good idea to kiss anything anymore—except my wife.

June 23, 2020

I love spending time with my family after an assignment. It helps me unwind again. I really love spending time with Sandra every day. I was spoiled from the very first time we met. She made sure I was happy in every aspect of our relationship. I always have been told if you keep a happy wife, you have a happy life. It helps knowing my wife loves me more than I can ever imagine. I truly feel like the luckiest man on the planet.

We are bikers. We do bicycles (mountain bikes, road bikes, etc.) like many Coloradans. But we ride motorcycles too. It's one of our favorite things to do after a long hard assignment away any time of year. Today we headed through Gunnison and Montrose, riding through the Blue Mesa—absolutely gorgeous blue lake. Then we passed through the Black Hills—black as coal mountain range. We rode to the city of Ouray, also known as the Switzerland of America. The highway is known for its extraordinary red rocks, mountain ridges, waterfalls, and a lot of heavenly beauty you can only find in Colorado. The town is full of nice friendly locals who are always willing to tell you how many things you can do for excitement and adventure. There is this amazing ice climbing wall, which of course we couldn't see in the summertime. I do lots of things Coloradans do, but I am not interested in climbing a wall of ice. That is worse than asking me to go swim in the ocean without a life vest—not me!

June 25, 2020

Sandra's daughter, Elise, had a birthday right before I came home. Since I missed it, we got together today for a celebration dinner. Elise is a paramedic and fire fighter with the department here. I always found that confusing. Don't paramedics ride in ambulances and fire fighters ride on the big red trucks? When a person calls 911, the dispatcher asks questions to figure out who is best to send on the call. Sometimes police are needed. Sometimes there is a fire and a truck is necessary. Most times, someone needs an ambulance. In many cities, the ambulance is part of the hospital, but they could also be an independent company. Here, the ambulance is part of the fire department and every fire fighter is cross-trained as an EMT or paramedic. Sometimes Elise is scheduled as a fire fighter on the truck and sometimes she is the medic on the ambulance.

EMS workers practice for every possible disaster, so they are ready if and when the time comes. They have always been the ones to run to disasters such as anthrax scares, Ebola outbreaks, or mass shootings while everyone else is running away. It was amazing to hear about their organized COVID preparation and response, not just in Denver, but on a national level.

Even though the EMS service does not have a "national voice," they quickly organized as one team when the crisis started in March to be able to learn from one another. EMS workers have lived up to their reputation of being willing and able to rise up to the unsurmountable challenges we have seen during this COVID disaster with professionalism and skill.

Top EMS leaders across the entire country met every week to share what they learned and took the best information back to their states. Each group evaluated what did and didn't work, along with ways to improve. They reviewed how often and when to test first responders, discussed where they should be in the vaccination order, and made certain they had enough PPE to do their jobs and stay safe. This group was unified.

One of the first adjustments EMS made was to change how they responded to 911 calls. If the patient could safely walk, they were asked to go outside to meet the crew. If that wasn't possible, they would send in just the number of people who were absolutely necessary based on the information the caller gave. Usually, it was only one person dressed in full hazmat gear going into the possible coronavirus space. Those guidelines helped limit exposure to the rest of the very small team. If more people were needed, they radioed for help. In the end, they did what was necessary at that time. The patient's safety always came before their own.

I have seen medical communities across the country become overwhelmed so fast they could not calmly organize and coordinate to be able to work together as one unit. We were hoping for some sort of national leadership that would bring experts together, gather information, and make recommendations for all of us to follow.

Each individual hospital or medical school (or group) tried to work together in their individual environments. They read what they could and made their own decisions on treatments and ways to handle the surge. Sandra managed doctors in twenty-six states across the country. She saw how every state was doing their own thing and no one had the time or the national platform to coordinate. Everyone was trying to re-invent the wheel without learning what not to do by other people's failures. We couldn't take advantage of other people's successes and use that as a best practice. Hospitals in the Northeast did things differently than those in the South, and the West coast had their own preferences also.

Doctors and nurses were in short supply. If they were taken out of commission, patients would not be able to get care. Why couldn't our government take control early in this crisis with a legitimate COVID task force using professional guidance from the CDC, respected physicians, and top scientists to formulate a coordinated plan for our hospitals to follow early in this crisis?

I wish I could make a video to send to all the hospitals in every state showing them the benefit of extension tubing for the IV pumps and how it saves nurses from going into the rooms dozens of times per day. I would love to show all the nurses how to prone a patient with only one person to help, instead of waiting for additional people who may not come. But it would be one video by one nurse. Who would watch it? How would it be distributed to every hospital in our nation without national leadership? How long is it going to take for us to unite as a medical community?

June 29, 2020

All these Black Lives Matter protests led to reform. In Mississippi, the legislature passed a bill to remove the Confederate symbol from the state flag. This is a remarkable change in the state where I was born and raised. Every time I looked at that flag, I was reminded my ancestors did not have a choice where they lived or what they did as a profession. Living with their family was not their choice to make. All those decisions were made by the person who owned them. Many positive changes have happened since then, but it will take a lot more than a signed decree to remove those same hate symbols from front porches and truck tailgates on the streets of Mississippi. If we come together for a common purpose, accept our differences, along with appreciating our strengths, we could heal this social wound of discrimination.

June 30, 2020

	COVID CASES		COVID DEATHS	
JAN	Global 12,308	US 1	Global 265	US 0
FEB	Global 86,471	US 60	Global 2,978	US 0
MAR	Global 889,005	US 149,378	Global 45,236	US 5,210
APR	Global 3,482,232	US 1,086,625	Global 238,993	US 62,955
MAY	Global 6,515,313	US 1,856,560	Global 382,743	US 108,439
JUN	Global 10,575,194	US 2,762,809	Global 526,357	US 129,710

July 1, 2020

I came home from New York less than two weeks ago completely drained. It's taken me longer to decompress. Under normal conditions, working in the ICU with the sickest of the sick is a grueling task. COVID placed this job in a whole new dimension. The medical journals reported overall ICU mortality estimated in the beginning of this crisis to be about 60%. They also stated this has improved as we learned more about this disease with current death rates at 43%.

This was not consistent with what I was seeing. The sheer volume of patients in the ICU in the Northeast was staggering. In busier ICUs, I saw much higher death rates than these reports. If a small hospital had only a handful of intubated patients, the nurses could manage that workload and get everything done that the patient needed in a day. I am sure this would affect whether that patient did well or not. If you average 90% death rate with 29%, the overall ICU mortality result is 60%. What I am saying is, the reported averages are probably correct taking into account every hospital and every ICU in the United States. But there is a lot more to the story than just that number.

Since there was no clear coordinated effort for treatment protocols, every school of medicine or major hospital published their own version of what to do and what to give a decompensated coronavirus patient. Doctors read this article or that one and had to figure out which treatment plan was most commonly used and hope for success.

The medical community didn't have the time to perform double-blind scientific studies or publish a review of previous cases for learning. There was no time because the virus came on so quickly. We all were thrown in the trenches, doing the best we could for this patient dying in front of us at that very moment. Many hospitals didn't have doctors with personal experience with some effective techniques, like proning for example. I'm sure all these things affected the mortality variation I am seeing across the country from what is reported in the media.

July 2, 2020

It felt like I was home for a day, but it was almost time to get back to work. Before I left, I had to ride to a little mountain town to get my nature fix. Sandra and I love to go to the Switchback Smokehouse where they have the best melt-in-your-mouth smoked duck and salmon. They have enough outside eating spread far apart, so if someone coughed or if the wind blew the disease would unlikely infect us. We made sure to get a table in the corner far from anyone else and wore our masks right up until our food came to our table. We would be more comfortable with take-out, but on our motorcycles that was impossible.

Back on the bikes there was nothing like feeling the wind wrap around my naked arms riding on a warm summer day right before dusk. The mountain wind was cool mixed with the heat from the road and it hugged me like a warm blanket on a cold winter morning. People who ride motorcycles experience something unique that you will only understand if you actually experience it yourself. The air with changes in ambient temperature—cold, hot, warm, to just right as we rode through the twisty turns and switch backs on mountain roads brought different smells in the air; wood from fireplaces, water from the lakes, rain that we hoped didn't come our way, and even there was dead roadkill. All of these sensations at once reminded me of a dog hanging out of a car window with its tongue flapping in the wind trying to capture it all.

July 3, 2020

I left home again today for the next deployment. It was a war. It was a deployment. As a traveler, I tried to schedule my shifts excluding important holidays, so I could spend every celebration at home with my family. This year would be different. I'd miss the Fourth of July, but there was no time. I was now restless with the urgency to get back to work.

The airport was very busy on the day I flew back to New York to get my car. After being off for a couple of weeks in beautiful Colorado, I dreaded going again to the big city. Being in the airport reminded me of the hustle and bustle rat race. Thankfully, most of the folks around Denver listen to the rules. Inside the airport it was a different story. I cringed when I saw folks had their masks pulled down under their noses barely covering their mouths. Air comes into the nose, similar to the mouth, and so can coronavirus. I saw children not wearing masks. Some parents apparently thought their kids must have some superhuman disease fighting power.

The security line was short, probably due to the fact less people were traveling these days. I was literally groped and searched, which happens each time I fly. My physician wife told me it is because my muscles are so dense they set off the machine every single time. I don't know if that's true, but she's usually right. Security searched my backpack, but only found my champagne toast scented candle I bring to get my travel room to smell like home. After I was released, I slipped on my shoes and belt and headed to the underground train that goes to the terminal.

The train can get very crowded at times and it was especially so today. It seemed weird at first because so few people are traveling, and then I realized they must have adjusted the running schedule to compensate. Statistically, out of all these folks, at least five or six probably have coronavirus. I had my head turned, almost smashing my face into the window attempting to get out of others' personal space and tried not to breathe the air. We finally came to the terminal and everyone moved simultaneously, like a giant mudslide after a torrential rain.

I headed up the escalator and while I walked to the terminal, I noticed people in restaurants not wearing masks sitting right next to one another—like things were normal in this world. I get they have to eat, but don't these folks know there's a pandemic going on? To tune it out, I listened to my Beats. I was in a zone, but still aware of my surroundings. It was early and I didn't have to rush, but I was relieved to arrive at the gate. I never like feeling that I could miss my flight.

Once we boarded, several people thought they could be sneaky and pulled their masks down under their noses. The flight attendants had to tell them to put their masks on correctly or they would be asked to leave the plane. I liked that they were so strict! But we hadn't even left the tarmac yet and people were already trying to bend the rules. I was glad to have an N95 and a cloth mask on top. Double protection.

Still, I felt uncomfortable the entire flight back to New York. As we approached the Big Apple, I stared over the endless shimmering of city lights as far as my eyes would allow. How could so many people be jammed pack in such a small area? Knowing I was about to land made me have a hankering for the best pizza on this planet. Since I was here for a few short hours before my drive to Florida, there was only one option for my dessert tonight; there is a reason they put the word New York in front of cheesecake.

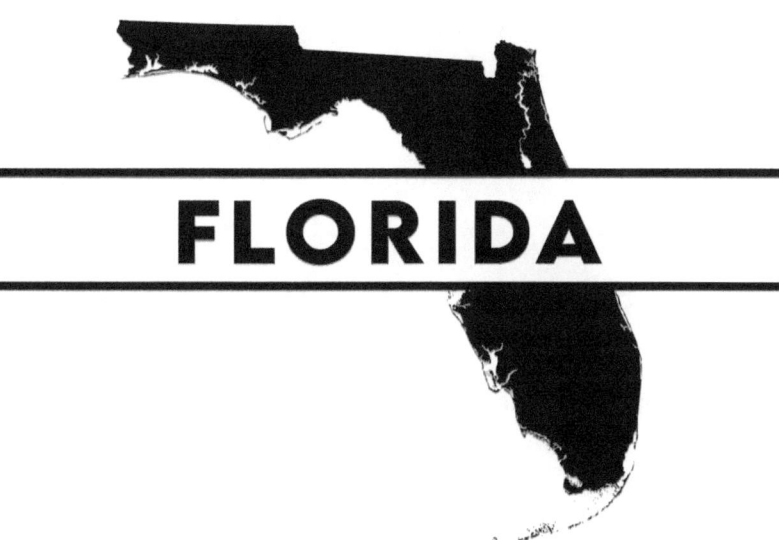

July 4, 2020

I started my drive early in the morning to Miami for my next assignment that would start in a couple of days. I felt rested despite arriving the night before with little time to relax.

On the drive south, it was shocking to see the lax attitudes of social distancing and non-compliance for mask wearing of the general public. When I stopped for gas or food, I rarely saw anyone wearing a mask. It did vary slightly state to state, but it was all bad. The worst states for not adhering to CDC recommendations started from Virginia all the way through Georgia. It wasn't until at the state line of Florida when I started to see more people wearing masks.

July 6, 2020

Security escorted four other nurses and me to the orientation area on my first day at work. The hospital was in a bad part of town, but I was not here to sight-see. Hospital orientation usually lasting five days was reduced to one for orientation and another for computer training. At the end of the second day, we were taken from department to department as an introduction, to see what we could expect. Crazy how they squeezed it all in to get us functioning enough to work the units this quickly. The hospital was overflowing, and my stomach started to churn. People were running around trying to get things done and it was plain to see how the staff was stressed to the max. Soon I discovered this overwhelmed hospital was losing nurses by the handfuls, every day. The hospital hired fifteen nurses who were supposed to start orientation with me. Only five of us showed up and actually started working. The others ran for the proverbial hills before Day One.

Usually, a hospital has a charge nurse on every unit and a nurse manager to oversee the charge nurses. In this hospital, the upper administration was trying to do administrative duties like hiring and firing, orienting travel nurses like me, while also functioning as managers for the Medical Units and all the ICUs. The lack of leadership on the floor affected the morale of the workers, resulting in low employee satisfaction and high turnover. I saw these similar short-staffed situations across the country.

The admission surges from this outbreak were dramatically increasing the workload for nurses, cracking wide open this already stressed situation. This hospital would greatly benefit in investing in managers and extension tubing like the New York facility. Even though I discussed it with them, I can imagine it would be hard to take the word of one travel nurse. If only we had a coordinated national team, we could get through this crisis easier.

July 11, 2020

There was a lot of talk in the news about this being an election year and how with COVID, political rallies were really unsafe. Some candidates held rallies outdoors or virtually to comply with social distancing. Others were held with no regard for COVID precautions. These rallies seemed pointless in a pandemic. The attendance numbers were low compared to any other year and the people who attended were already supporters of their candidate. They did not need convincing anyway.

The one in New Hampshire was interesting to me because local Republicans wanted the rally postponed or cancelled to allow the state to safely recover from the recent COVID surge. The Republican President was insisting on holding it anyway. It turned out Mother Nature helped with that decision. A tropical storm blew in and the rally couldn't proceed.

July 15, 2020

This very busy day in the ICU was coming to an end after twelve long hours. I was wrapping up my charting and giving report to the on-coming nurse when I was approached by the Director of the Emergency Department. He stood in front of me with his hands clasped as if praying and asked, "Can you please stay longer and fill in as the Emergency Room Charge Nurse?"

I looked at him in disbelief as his eyes continued to plead. I was a traveler, assigned to the ICU in a very busy hospital, and he wanted me to be in charge of the ED! I'd been here less than two weeks. I have worked in this ED as a float nurse maybe three or four times, but I didn't know all the duties and responsibilities of a Charge Nurse for this facility. I took a deep breath and saw his personal desperation.

"Yes, I'm happy to help y'all. I'll do it," I said. Of course, I couldn't leave that man hanging. This day was getting longer and longer by the minute. I knew the ED was short staffed by at least five nurses. There were sixty-eight patients in a thirty-four bed ED with forty more patients in the waiting room. The line for registration was out the door. How was I going to do this? I needed help.

Emilio and Chad were also finishing their twelve-hour shifts and are great ICU nurses, along with being fantastic work horses. They could help me as "runners" doing tasks such as starting IVs, hanging medications, participating in code blues—whatever was needed. This could work.

I showed up at shift change to a room of oncoming nurses. They already knew I was designated as Charge and most were relieved. One nurse was obviously put out that even after I already worked a hectic twelve-hour shift, I was chosen to lead this team tonight. I knew I had to quickly take control to not have dissenters in the ranks. I asked him, "I see you have a problem with me being Charge. Would you like to step up and do this instead of me?"

The entire room got suddenly quiet and they looked at us. He paused, and slowly looked around, then answered, "I don't have a problem with you."

I looked at everyone and said, "I know it is unusual to have a traveler as Charge, and I will not let you down. And I don't want you to let me down, either. As a reward for all your hard work and support tonight, I will buy everyone pizza and chicken wings for supper!" The mood instantly changed. With the team behind me, we would have a great night.

My first challenge this evening was managing a mother who brought her three-month-old into the emergency room. After the physician examined the baby, he felt the child's injuries were suspicious for sexual abuse. My first task was to get law enforcement involved. I went to the patient's room to get some information—and the mother had fled with the child before the police could arrive! I had no idea what I was supposed to do next. I had never been in this unusual situation before. I looked up the patient's address in the computer and gave it to the cops. It was better for them to take it from here because the patient was no longer on the hospital premises, and there were many other fires to handle.

One of the doctors on shift was frazzled and clearly exhausted by the tremendous number of patients he had seen. I knew his day was just as challenging as mine. His critical COVID patient ended up coding after hours and hours of treatment, and died. The doc slumped in his chair at the desk to complete his charts. Only then did he realize all of his notes on every patient he had seen during the day with much detailed descriptions of what was done and what was given vanished into cyberspace. He called IT and they could not recover any documentation he wrote or any dictations from his shift. The doc looked up at me, grabbed his bag and said, "Fuck this shit. I am tired of this," and walked out. He quit his job right then and there.

A few days earlier, a COVID-positive patient with psychiatric issues was admitted, but he had to stay in a non-private bay in the ED because there were no hospital rooms available. This patient had become increasingly agitated and almost unmanageable. He wanted to leave tonight. As Charge, I knew I needed to try my best to resolve his concerns, so he would remain in the hospital for his necessary treatments.

With a little calm questioning about why he was upset, I found out he had been trying for two days to get someone to help him charge his dead phone. He knew his wife and daughter were worried about him. I looked at his cell and saw he needed the same charger I use. Such an easy fix! I walked out to my car, got my cord, and the guy started smiling again.

He finally confessed that he had been drinking, passed out on a sidewalk, and was brought to this hospital without his family knowing anything. After his phone charged, I called his wife (nobody memorizes phone numbers anymore). She started crying immediately when I told her who I was, and that we had her husband safe and sound. They thought he was dead.

Just as soon as I got this guy settled, I heard a commotion in the ambulance bay entrance. A forty-five-year-old drunk woman was yelling, cussing, and trying to leave the hospital without permission, even though she was in the custody of three security officers. She caused a pretty serious accident and was arrested for DUI. On the initial evaluation, the medical team was concerned she might have a neck injury. She had abrasions on the left side of her head and face, as well as shards of glass in her hair. All this was evidence she hit her head hard enough on the driver's side window to break it. One of the officers reported when they arrived at the intersection, she was confused and not answering questions appropriately. She couldn't tell them what happened and couldn't follow directions. We immediately placed a cervical collar on her while waiting to get a CAT scan, looking for a fractured vertebra.

Now things were starting to intensify. She seemed barely coherent and out of her mind, ranting and raving about suing anyone who touched her as she ripped off her neck brace. She was obviously drunk and irrational while stumbling around, bumping into all the equipment trying to get out of the door. The police, a doctor, and a nurse were trying to coax her to get back in the room, to lay on the gurney and secure her neck collar again in place.

As we were struggling to keep the patient safe, the officers told us what they had learned from her family. Her sister had died from COVID and the funeral was today. To make matters worse, she was an alcoholic and did not hesitate to overindulge in her grief. The smell of alcohol oozed out of her skin and as we could have predicted, her BAL (blood alcohol level) was off the charts. She drove recklessly when she left the funeral and got T-boned on the driver's side.

I got right in front of her and addressed her directly, "How can I help you? What can I do to make you want to stay? We are very concerned that you might have a broken neck and could end up paralyzed if you don't put that brace back on."

"All I want is some fuckin' water!" she yelled, turning her head looking around the room. If her neck was fractured, she really could make things horribly worse by moving around like this.

"Okay, that is really easy. If I get you some water right now, will you get back in bed for me?"

She looked me up and down with her half-closed drunken eyes and smiled at me with her gaping split lower lip dripping blood. She said, "I ain't nevah seen a nurse that looked like you. I'll do whatevah you say." Then she turned around and staggered back into bed. I got her some food and water and asked the doc to order some Ativan as an anxiety medication to hopefully keep her calm. She became a different person, smiling and happy. I am so thankful we were successful in deescalating this situation and were able to get her neck brace secured in place. The CT scan results showed two fractured vertebrae at C4 and C5. She really could have ended up paralyzed if she had slipped and fallen on the floor. Even just turning her head quickly could have done her in.

July 21, 2020

I worked in the ED a few days, then back to the ICU. Today, I was assigned a woman on BiPAP who only spoke Spanish. She was anxious and yanked off her life saving mask. Immediately she turned blue and almost passed out. This occurred time and time again. She was agitated and couldn't communicate well due to the language barrier and the breathing machine. She needed this high level of oxygen to stay alive.

As a last effort before she potentially coded, I asked the doc to try High Flow oxygen, which is less claustrophobic feeling than BiPAP. The High Flow method doesn't work as well as BiPAP, but it would be better than her not wearing any mask at all. I stumbled with the little Spanish I know and got her to try it, telling her, "Es mejor!" (It is better!) "No da miedo!" (It is not scary!) Finally, she let me put this nasal cannula on her and her oxygen saturation rose to 88%, holding steady. It wasn't perfect, but it would do. I got her a small dose of Ativan to calm her nerves and she settled in for the night. She was a nice lady in a terrible situation.

July 23, 2020

At the start of my busy shift, a thirty-six-year-old Black American male patient came into the emergency room for shortness of breath and difficulty breathing related to COVID. This patient had a rapid coronavirus test while out in the ambulance bay which came back positive. He weighed 550 pounds and could barely fit on the ambulance gurney. Most of the gurneys have a weight limit of 500 pounds. Unfortunately, neither the ambulance nor the hospital had the 700-pound maximum weight version.

As we wheeled him off the ambulance in the bay, the gurney broke, and the patient started to fall. Fortunately, the six staff members who were there helped lower him to the ground in a controlled fashion, preventing him from getting hurt. There were several male nurses (me included) who together thought we were capable of picking him up to place him on a bariatric bed. We were mistaken. Most hospitals have what is called a Hoyer Lift. It also has a weight limit, which he exceeded. The charge nurse had to call the fire department that had some kind of device which was successful in getting the patient safely into the bed. Keep in mind, this patient was short of breath during this entire ordeal.

I finally was able to get his vital signs, which included an oxygen saturation that read 78% on 15 liters non-rebreather. The non-rebreather is a way we administer oxygen to a patient as a final effort before having to resort to more aggressive means.

He needed the more aggressive means of oxygenation, which is intubation. It sounds really simple, to put a tube down someone's throat into their lungs to help them breathe. Well, this one wasn't so simple. When people are significantly overweight, the excess tissue around the neck and face make the intubation procedure extremely difficult. Sometimes it is not successful. During this process, it is necessary to tilt the head far back and open the mouth as wide as possible. This guy had no neck, and his mouth could not open more than about an inch. How was the doc going to be able to see to put the tube in the right place?

The doc took one look at this patient's mouth and thought the same thing. He hurried to the next room and brought back an intubation video machine. It has a light and camera at the end of the intubating plastic "blade." Everyone in the room could see the vocal chords as clear as crystal. The doc made it look so easy as he slid that tube right between the vocal chords into the lungs. Now the patient started getting the oxygen he needed and his sats started to rise.

His family members called to check up on him and I spoke with his wife. She said his shortness of breath started two days prior to him coming to the ER. He was morbidly obese and had a history of diabetes, high blood pressure, high cholesterol, and kidney disease, and smoked two packs of cigarettes per day for many years. I knew from his medical history and since he was already intubated, the outcome of his visit was not in his favor.

I asked his wife, "Where do you think he came in contact with the virus?"

She said, "We were at a party on the Friday before last with about forty people. We found out afterward that two people there were positive with the virus. None of us wore masks."

We started the usual coronavirus regime with antivirals, antibiotics, steroids, and blood thinners. This patient was admitted to ICU and would be assigned a room as soon as one was available. My ED shift ended for the evening. I went to my room to get a few hours of sleep before returning the next day.

The following day, I was assigned to ICU, and guess who was my patient? I felt so sorry for him and his family. He had four children between the ages of three and ten. I could hear the kids in the background as I spoke with his wife. They kept asking, "When is Daddy coming home?"

She wanted me to tell her he was doing better since his admission yesterday, but I had to tell her the truth. He actually coded once during the night. They were able to bring him back, but his kidneys were failing. He was maxed out on all the medications we could give him for sedation, and his blood pressure was dropping. Then he started having rectal bleeding and bloody secretions from his sputum when we suctioned him.

I was on the phone with his wife when I looked at the patient's monitor and saw his heart rate dropping to 50s, then 40s, then 30s. I dropped the phone, ran into his room, and pushed the code blue button. As I started CPR, the team responded rapidly to assist in what was another long stressful and unforgettable experience. We worked on this guy for 45 minutes before the physician called it. "Time of death, 1535."

When I sat down to chart what happened over the last hour, I realized the phone was off the hook and lying on the table. His wife was still holding all this time. I told her that I would have her speak with the resident who was standing right next to me. The doctor took the phone and told the wife, "I'm very sorry, ma'am. Your husband did not make it. We did all we could do." I heard her weeping on the phone, with her children in the background asking her, "What's wrong Mom?" I walked away, went back into the patient's room, and held his hand as I prayed for him and his family.

Once I exited the room, another code blue was called on my unit across the hall. I ran to assist my co-workers. Today we had another forty code blues in the hospital. I felt shell shocked and devastated with too much death and most of it preventable.

July 26, 2020

On my lunch break I called Sandra. She told me that a couple of days ago her sister was waiting for Hurricane Douglas in Hawai'i. Ja-ne is a caregiver for her adopted mother, Moana. They live by themselves in a small house and have been pretty much isolated since March. To prepare for the hurricane, she dragged in everything from outside and set up lanterns and solar lights all over the house because Moana is afraid of the dark. She put extra water in containers and cooked a whole lot of food to last a while and also to share. If the hurricane hit, they wouldn't have electricity for a long time. Ja-ne prepared non-stop for two days and then on the big day, she waited and waited and waited. At the last minute, Douglas scooted past the island. It was so close, people photographed it from shore. Now everything had to go back in its regular place. The 93-year-old was upset because they ran out of homemade ice cream, which is her only priority at this point in her life. And yesterday in Texas, Sandra's father geared for Hurricane Hannah. I can't imagine what's going to come up next.

July 27, 2020

I realized there were some nurses I hadn't seen lately. I asked my co-worker if those missing nurses were reassigned to a sister hospital in the area. She laughed sarcastically and said I was naïve. Then she told me over one hundred nurses have quit this hospital within the last month, half of them employed staff and the other half short term travel nurses. That is just incredible! I am certainly aware of the new demands on nurses during this COVID crisis. It has exceeded what is usual and customary. The normal nurse to patient ratio in an ICU is 1:1 or 1:2. Now we were 1:3 and sometimes 1:4. These ICU patients took so much time and energy I guess these nurses eventually reached their breaking point and quit. Just like that doctor who quit in the ER after the computer lost all his notes.

Even under normal non-COVID circumstances, when I am assigned to the same unit day after day, it is much easier to take care of someone I already know. It makes it easier to predict what patients may need. Communication is also much faster when I know their hand signals and reactions. It makes my day better and it is professionally satisfying to know I'm doing everything I can to help them recover.

I asked to get reassigned to a lady I took care of a couple of days ago. When I went into her room, she smiled at me. She was nice and tried to help me improve my "Span-glish" in between long pauses to catch her breath. When I was starting to do my assessment of her legs, I pulled back the sheet. Black toes! She had gangrene. Her legs were swollen with blisters everywhere. Why did this happen in just a short time?! I have seen this in septic ICU patients with low blood pressure when they require strong medications to push the blood pressure up. These meds work by squeezing the little blood vessels in the fingers and toes, far away from the heart to redirect the blood to the core and vital organs. I looked in her chart and found we never used these drugs on this woman because her pressure was always normal. This lady's black toes were not a side-effect of any medication. This must have been all COVID. It was such an oxymoron how coronavirus could cause bloody mucous in the lungs and rectal bleeding, then cause clotting in the tiny vessels in the toes or fingers. She would lose her toes due to this damn coronavirus. I hope that would be all she would lose from this infection. We had to get her back on BiPAP to optimize the oxygen in her blood, or she could lose her feet, or even her legs, or maybe her life.

The doc ordered a Precedex drip to try to keep her calm enough to tolerate BiPAP again. Eventually, she was one of the lucky ones who improved enough to get out of the ICU. I am certain it will take months before she would be able to be discharged to rehab. Then more months before she could go home to care for herself. This experience has been life changing, not just for her, but for her entire family and friends who love her. Coronavirus is affecting billions more than just the sick—directly or indirectly, every human in existence is touched by this disease.

July 31, 2020

	COVID CASES		COVID DEATHS	
JAN	Global 12,308	US 1	Global 265	US 0
FEB	Global 86,471	US 60	Global 2,978	US 0
MAR	Global 889,005	US 149,378	Global 45,236	US 5,210
APR	Global 3,482,232	US 1,086,625	Global 238,993	US 62,955
MAY	Global 6,515,313	US 1,856,560	Global 382,743	US 108,439
JUN	Global 10,575,194	US 2,762,809	Global 526,357	US 129,710
JUL	Global 17,627,792	US 4,708,945	Global 694,078	US 157,386

August 1, 2020

My daily routine here was to go to the staffing office every morning to get my assignment for the day and get my rationed PPE. With shortages seen in this pandemic, our hospital was tightly regulating supplies, in hopes we didn't run out. In a perfect world, every healthcare worker would wear a new N95 mask for each patient every day. In this COVID world, we had to use the same mask all day long, day after day, knowing the level of protection went down the longer it was used. We would try to keep it clean by wearing a fresh surgical mask on top that would be discarded after one use. They would give us a new N95 only if the straps were broken or it was visibly soiled, no matter how many days we had already worn it.

Since I was working over twelve hours every single day, there was zero chance I could order my own masks online.

And with all the shortages, I doubt I would have been able to buy them anyway.

We also were given only one disposable gown to use for the entire day for each of our patients. These are paper or plastic gowns and are supposed to be used once and thrown away when we leave the room. Now after treating a patient, we were expected to clean our gown with sanitizing wipes and leave it on a hook just outside the door in the hall. There was no other place to put it. How could any of this be safe infection control practices?

In New York, we lined up every morning for a new mask and there were carts with plenty of disposable gowns outside of each room. I felt safer working in New York than I do here. I am worried I could catch this virus even though I am super careful.

Another important nursing issue that changed with COVID is scanning medications before giving them to a patient. Every patient gets an identification armband on admission listing their name, DOB, medical record number, and hospital account number. The armband has a barcode that is scanned every time a medication is scheduled to be administered. This process helps prevent the error of accidentally giving a drug to the wrong person. But this requires the computer to be in the room next to the patient.

In small hospitals, they may have enough computers to leave one in every room, but in larger hospitals or in makeshift COVID units not originally intended for patient care, there may not be a computer close enough or one that can be dedicated to a specific patient. We certainly cannot take the same computer in and out of the coronavirus infected area, then back to the nurse's station to do our work. There is no way to safely scan armbands before giving meds in this pandemic.

We were seeing so many sick patients being admitted and placed on ventilators, they converted the regular Medical floor to an ICU. The semi-private rooms usually housing two patients now are stuffed with four critically ill people on vents. At first, this may sound logical, but it proved to be very problematic. The Medical Unit is not set up for critical conditions. ICU patients require constant tracking, and these rooms aren't equipped with the proper machines to monitor blood pressure, pulse, oxygen saturations, and heart rhythm. We borrowed portable monitors from sister hospitals which did not solve our problem. The nurses' station is not situated to be able to maintain visual contact with these intubated patients. Even if the doors are open (which isn't a good idea with COVID-positive patients), the beds are positioned in such a way the nurse has to walk in the door to see how the patients are doing. We started sitting in the hallway outside the open rooms to try to keep our eye on the patients, and also to be in close proximity to be able to respond quickly to their constantly changing conditions.

The hospital now is a sea of perpetual disorganization. Code blues are constantly called overhead. Usually, there is a code team to respond to the emergency. In the ICU, we almost never see the code team here because they are always busy with another urgent situation. Many times, it is just another nurse and me doing CPR for about ten minutes before a physician would be free to be able to respond to our call for help. This hospital is fortunate to have a physician residency program. They may not know everything yet, but they are in training and can provide another set of hands to do the work.

August 6, 2020

Today I took care of a thirty-six-year-old lady weighing 750 pounds with diabetes and COVID who was on a ventilator. She was likely going to die. We had her on all the ICU drips: remdesivir and plasma, sedation meds to help her not feel the tube down her throat, paralytics to help her not fight the breathing machine, blood thinners, and IV fluids.

To prevent her from getting skin breakdown from constant moisture, we had to put in a urinary catheter. This may seem easy, but her size made this routine task problematic. It took seven of us to get this done. Two people held each leg in position, two people on each side held back her pannus with a large sheet, and one person tried to insert the catheter. It did not work at first, but we kept trying. Finally, on the fourth attempt and twenty minutes later, we were successful.

On a daily basis, I spoke with her twin sister. I learned the entire household caught the virus from their sixteen-year-old brother who went to a party without paying attention to proper protocol. He brought this infection home to his entire family.

After three weeks of treatment in the ICU on a ventilator, she started declining, and we called a code blue. We coded her four times that day. Towards the end, I relayed messages to my patient from her sister telling her encouraging words. "You are the strongest person I know, and we will continue to pray for you, sister. I know you will get better." Even though she was sedated and on the respirator, I spoke softly in her ear. She was a Christian woman who went to church regularly. I felt compelled to support her with a prayer and sang a hymn to her in hopes she heard these positive messages. Within two weeks her grandmother, mother, and my patient died, all in the same hospital. This was devastating to the family. Worst of all it could have been completely prevented.

August 10, 2020

Here, the mortality of a COVID ICU patient on a breathing machine was usually over 90%. We had better averages in the northeast. There were many factors that could contribute to this difference. Not understanding how to safely prone patients is one issue. The lack of adequate staff and the grossly overfilled hospital also contributed to why we could not do all the things every patient needed. Nurse fatigue also caused mistakes, like connecting the oxygen tube on the ventilator to the normal air port on the wall. Thankfully, that particular error was caught by the respiratory therapy tech before the patient had issues. Maybe there was no time to suction the lungs of one patient because the other one was coding. Another patient was seizing, so you left the room where the repositioning and breathing treatments were due. All these things affected whether the patients got better or not.

August 14, 2020

In this crisis, the patient usually progresses from a nasal canula to a face mask, then a non-rebreather mask, and then this ventilated support machine like the CPAP or BiPAP machine. At this point, the patients have air hunger with no relief. They are suffocating and feeling the reality that death is near. Try putting your head under water as long as you possibly can, blowing out your air slowly until you are completely out. Then stay there a little longer. When you eventually come up and get a big breath of fresh air, it is such relief. Well, this is the only wish these patients have right now. They would do anything to be able to breathe again. What I have seen since March was once my patients needed this necessary piece of equipment, their lives were starting to circle the drain. There would not be much time to make a difference.

One consistent aspect I see is coronavirus patients in the hospital become extremely weak. Those on BiPAP or those who are able to improve and get off the ventilator are aware of how sick and debilitated they really have become. These patients can't do anything for themselves without help. Since they haven't stood on their own two legs for several weeks, they cannot walk themselves to the bathroom. Some are so weak they are unable to grasp a fork and lift it to their mouths. And they are alone. They haven't seen their families since they arrived here and aren't able to have visitors. They will have a long rehab road to recovery, but at least they have their lives.

August 17, 2020

One common theme I saw from state to state during this disaster was how doctors are struggling to find good ways to treat coronavirus. Usually, they are confident in handling standard medical issues. They have years of experience with normal diagnoses. This tragedy is challenging physicians, both mentally and physically. They are racing to find appropriate treatments that will work before each patient dies.

First, we had hopes in using hydroxychloroquine with azithromycin. This seemed to work initially, but with many trials, we saw no reduction in mortality at all. In fact, there were numerous reports of cardiac issues caused by this regimen. Now, our hopes are with remdesivir, which seems promising. We also have convalescent plasma and new drugs in Phase 3 trials.

Other than medications, doctors are trying to figure out the best settings for respirators for this disease. Patients are requiring very high pressures to maintain their oxygen levels, but these high pressures tend to also cause trauma to their lungs.

A resident came in to evaluate my patient with COVID and increased the ventilator rate to 60 with PEEP pressure of 40. Normally for non-COVID issues, patients are on respiration rates between 12-25 breaths per minute and additional PEEP pressure of 5-10. These lower settings are not working for the COVID patients intubated on these vents. The doctors try higher settings in a last attempt to put more oxygen in the blood, which seems to work temporarily. Ultimately, the lungs cannot withstand that for very long. If we keep up with that high pressure treatment, the patient's lungs could tear and deflate causing them to need a chest tube, and the patient may also die. What else can the doctors do? It is truly an impossible situation.

August 18, 2020

In New York and New Jersey, the ICU patients were frequently pronated and repositioned to help their lungs oxygenate. There was a team whose sole job was to prone people. It took up their entire day. They worked with the nurse assigned to the patient, so I learned from them. I showed the staff here how to do this with just one other person instead of a team. This process required patience, otherwise all the tubes and lines could get caught and pulled out. The docs started utilizing this life-saving technique and I am hopeful it will help more patients here survive this fight.

One of the worst and most deadly complications I have seen from coronavirus is pneumonia. The pictures are really dramatic on CT scans. It looks like ground glass in the lungs. It is not actually glass inside the patient, but fluid and mucus from the infection trapped in the tiny spaces deep inside the lung tissue. This fluid has a lacy appearance that someone fifty years ago thought looked like ground-up glass, which led to that description. This infection is relentless in attacking all the little pockets of the lungs depositing thick bloody mucus preventing oxygen from crossing into the bloodstream. The mucus is hard to suction out and accumulates with gravity deep in the lungs. Proning moves the mucus around, which allows the pockets to clear out, giving oxygen a chance to get into the blood.

Another issue we are seeing with this infection is patients are tending to get blood clots even months after the person recovers. These clots are showing up as heart attacks, strokes, and gangrene fingers and toes. It is thought that COVID is causing an underlying inflammation that is leading to all this extra morbidity. This is why these blood thinners are used, but then the patients bleed from their rectum or lungs. Damned if we do, damned if we don't in this fight.

August 19, 2020

Today was physically the hardest code I can ever remember as a nurse. A 33-year-old Black man hurricane-partied with over twenty friends during the first weekend this month to celebrate Isaac. It was not a hurricane like Camille, Fredrick, or Katrina, but it still was a bad storm. We were lucky to avoid a direct hit. This young man was not the only positive case in the group, but this time it was no party in the hospital. Now he was in the ICU with me. Eight other folks in the group came here also. Unfortunately, two of them already died.

We worked on him for an entire hour. I am in pretty good shape, but due to his size and the amount of force we needed to push on his chest to do compressions, my triceps and forearms burned. Compression after compression. Even though we took turns, exhaustion was taking over all of us.

The specific doc who was the leader of this code wanted to work on him a little longer because the patient was young and a fighter. We would get a heartbeat or pulse from time to time during the hour we worked on him, but he would brady down to asystole. His heart was giving up and flatlining. We worked through the ACLS algorithm over and over. We went through three crash carts. Eventually we could not save him. This was an awful day, but most of my days in Miami were like this.

Code blues were still happening all the time. Sometimes it was my patient, sometimes it was another patient in a different

ICU. And it wasn't only one person, but entire families would get wiped out. I worked with doctors and nurses who have been personally affected by this atrocity. They saw their own relatives here. It's a rare occasion to see your loved one go through this kind of torture, the excruciating long drawn-out suffering of this virus, until they finally die. Some say death is a consolation, but seeing the torment and suffering will linger in my mind for years to come.

August 20, 2020

At the end of the day just before we changed shift, I got an admission from the ER. This guy was an illegal immigrant who didn't speak English at all. Everyone admitted these days was COVID-positive, and he was no exception. The first thing I noticed was that he was "tripoding." That expressive term is used when a patient sits on the edge of the bed, leans forward with both elbows on the table in a tripod configuration holding their chest up, struggling to breathe. There are a few things in medicine that would cause a patient to sit up like that—a bad lung issue like an asthma attack, or a bad heart issue like cardiac tamponade. This guy wasn't wheezing, so it had to be his heart. Cardiac tamponade is when fluid is building up in the sack around the heart and eventually the heart is strangled. The chambers cannot stretch out and open to fill with blood to be able to pump properly. His blood pressure started to drop. I knew this was a medical emergency. The next thing that would happen was the patient would die.

Immediately, I called the resident who said he would order a chest X-ray and cardiac ultrasound and call me later. I pushed for these tests to be done ASAP and after the results were in, I called the resident again. He told me to call the Cardiothoracic Surgeon because he was under water and couldn't be in two places at once. Usually, docs require that another doc call them to ask for a consultation, not the nurse. In this case, I didn't hesitate to call the CT Surgeon, who also told me he was too busy to come see the patient and it had to wait. I understood these doctors were busy and there were many other critical patients competing for their attention. But if they didn't see him now, I knew he would quickly deteriorate and that would be the end of him.

I took a deep breath and explained more details about this critical emergency. What this patient needed was to go to surgery or die. The surgeon took a second, but then realized this patient needed to come first. He called the OR team to get ready, and I called the resident. The patient was tiring by the minute and could not breathe adequately anymore. His oxygen was down to 68% and he needed to be sedated, put on the breathing machine, and get an operation. There wasn't much time. The surgeon showed up and we prepped the patient for surgery STAT.

Finally, some good news for a change; the operation was a success. The surgeon removed a whole liter of bloody fluid from around this patient's heart. It was like his heart was being strangled by a 1000cc COVID-liquid python. He lived to see another day. A week later, I was sad to hear he died.

August 21, 2020

Nutrition is important to help patients stay strong in fighting this infection. Families always ask us about tube feedings for their loved ones. Intubated patients on a ventilator routinely get liquid nutrition through a tube from their nose or mouth directly to their stomach. Patients on BiPAP usually shouldn't have tube feedings as the pressure from the machine can force air in the stomach, causing the patient to possibly vomit. The emesis then goes down in the lungs, worsening their condition. Nutrition given intravenously is not optimal either, as it is associated with a high risk of fungal infections in the bloodstream but it is sometimes necessary.

August 22, 2020

The patients with families are the lucky ones. They have someone who calls leaving personal messages of encouragement. We sometimes schedule audio or video chats for them. They usually end up crying before the conversation is over. At least they are happy tears because they finally are able to see each other and have some communication, even in a virtual setting. But at the same time, they are devastated because the patient cannot come home for months and it is far from certain they will survive this.

The unlucky ones are the half a million homeless people in America, many who are huddled in crowded shelters. This puts them at high risk of contracting this contagious viral infection. I read that the homeless who keep out of shelters and instead stay outside in parks or on beaches have a lower risk of getting sick. Some cities are reinventing how they provide for this population by opening convention centers as large dormitories with socially distant cots. Despite some limited outbreaks in a few shelters, isolation has helped keep the overwhelming majority from exposure.

When they come to the hospital, they don't have anyone calling with supportive and encouraging messages. Many feel awkward to be around people and have trouble communicating besides not being able to talk when they are on these life-saving machines. They do get support with the overworked nurses and staff who become the surrogate family for this unfortunate subset of our population. To work in a hospital normally taxes the emotions, but these incomparable times are pushing these boundaries past any limits.

August 23, 2020

There was a travel nurse on the news spreading bad things about a hospital in New York, saying that doctors were killing patients. She also brought up the point that physicians were negligent, placing non-COVID patients in rooms with those positive for this virus. We had patients in hallways and practically on top of each other. Here we would use hospital bunkbeds, if that were a thing. We couldn't transfer patients to another hospital as all the hospitals were well over their normal capacity and there was no room anywhere.

I know we tried to keep COVID patients isolated, but at this point, we were drowning and had been since March. We had to put four patients in a room set up for just two. An empty spot would be filled with a patient, regardless if they were with COVID or not. This was not optimal but was unfortunately necessary. I wonder if this trash-talking nurse really understood the horrible predicament all of us in healthcare were in. Maybe this is Mother Nature's way of culling our overcrowded human population. In Man versus Man, we could possibly reason to come to a conflict resolution. Man versus Nature is a whole different ball game. Mother Nature does not discriminate with anyone around the world, from celebrities to political leaders to bus drivers to farmers to mothers to executives. She touches everyone with her force.

Some healthcare workers think the grass is greener somewhere else and quit when the job gets tough. With COVID, our job is tough everywhere. My typical ICU load here was three very critical patients, each one demanding every moment of my day. For example, one room may take four hours to stabilize blood pressure or oxygen, give medications, titrate drips in response to their ever-changing vital signs, replace all the IV medication and tube feeding bags, empty urine collection and change rectal bags, bathe, and reposition the patient.

During this time, my second patient has cardiac tamponade needing to be sedated and put on a breathing machine for emergency surgery, while my third patient's sedative and paralytics for the ventilator are running out. My first patient's insulin bag is now empty, and her blood sugar is going up. While all of this is going on, I have to document every minute detail. We try to help each other when we get caught up, but there is usually no time left in the day. The other nurses are in the same position as me, juggling their own critical situations. I cannot provide this many critically ill patients with everything they need. None of us can. I feel like I am past the end of my rope.

The nursing staff are not the only ones feeling the surge crunch. Respiratory therapists are the ones responsible for the breathing machines, helping with lung suctioning, and a wide variety of other duties. There are only three RTs on shift for this entire hospital with over 500 patients and all patients in the ICU are COVID-positive. I saw an RT the other day and I told him to hang in there. The guy shook his head. He said, "Overwhelmed is an understatement. No matter how many hours in the day, I cannot do enough. So much suctioning, mouth care, and chest percussions. It's never enough. No matter how hard I work, the majority won't walk out of this ICU, but I can't stop because there is the chance that a few might make it." I didn't have words to answer, so I patted him on the shoulder, and we kept on going.

The nurses must help with the RT responsibilities because their plate is already overflowing. Unfortunately, we barely have time in the day to get all the urgent medications and treatments done on time, which leaves the routine repositioning and RT duties to fall to a lower priority. There is not enough staff anywhere in the hospital to care for the patients already admitted and hundreds more are coming into the ED every single day needing medical attention. I have worked twelve hours or more every day and had one day off out of all my time here. There was no relief when I returned to my hotel to rest. I felt guilty relaxing for a few hours because they needed me twenty-four hours a day.

August 26, 2020

My assignment was coming to an end. The hospital asked me to stay for another thirty days. While I wanted to stay, I was exhausted and needed to go home to my wife for a while. I missed her and our dogs, and of course our kids. On my long drive back to Colorado, I planned to stop off in Tampa to see my son Trevor and his family. He just had a new baby nine months ago and I have never met her.

On the road, my thoughts went to all my recent patients, and I wondered if I could have done more to save their lives. I also worried I could possibly bring coronavirus into my son's home. How could I truly feel safe when I had to work without new clean protective equipment day after day? We still don't know all there is to know about this disease. There are so many stories of entire families getting sick and dying from one virus carrier being careless, infecting everyone in the home. I couldn't do this to my own family.

There is a difference in protection with the various face coverings and masks people are wearing. Cloth masks worn in public are simple barriers that prevent most of the large spit droplets from leaving one's mouth and nose with speaking, coughing, or sneezing. These droplets can travel through the air to another person who is near. I read these cloth masks are not 100% effective, but they help reduce the spread of infections. People who wear masks in public are being thoughtful of the other person who could get sick from them. It has been common practice for years in many Asian countries for people to use a mask if they have a cold to not infect others.

I've used surgical masks throughout my career. I was surprised to find in my research they are less effective than cloth masks. They are thin barriers used in hospitals that loop behind the ears, holding them in place over the nose and mouth. They fit loosely on the face. These masks are designed to protect the wearer against large droplets, splashes, or sprays of body fluids that may occur in a normal hospital setting. They do not filter out tiny organisms such as coronavirus.

My wife told me early in March how the N95 mask was the safest to use. They were hard to get because they were expensive and in limited supply. I made sure I used them the entire time I was in the hospital and around anyone out in public. In those early days, the CDC and hospital guidelines were for hospital employees to wear surgical masks at their workstation, and the N95 only in COVID-positive rooms or around potentially COVID-positive patients. In the emergency room all hospital employees wore surgical masks. When a patient came in, it was not known if they were COVID-positive or not. Many ER workers became sick as they were not adequately protected. They should have been wearing N95s at all times since the beginning of this crisis.

The N95 mask has been around for a long time. This mask is used in many professions besides the medical field to filter small particles from entering the lungs. Building contractors and painters routinely use these masks and they are widely available. At least they used to be before the pandemic. It protects the wearer and other people close by and is the best mask to wear in this crisis. I read it can filter particles as small as 0.1-0.3 microns in diameter and up to 95% of airborne particles. COVID-19 is 0.06-1.4 microns, so even with this excellent mask, it is still not 100% protective.

Any mask, however, is not a substitute for social distancing. Social distancing is most important as the concentration of droplets carrying the enemy reduces drastically after about six to ten feet. So, if you are wearing a mask and keeping ten feet away, the chances are great that you will not get sick.

I wore the N95 mask everywhere in Miami, in the hospital, and in public places. I also stayed socially distant as much as the situation allowed. In the hospital, I wore extra layers of protection when taking care of COVID patients, so I felt pretty confident I was not one of those carriers.

Once I arrived in Tampa, I got a rapid coronavirus test (my sixth test since this all began) which was again negative. Even with this test, I could be early in the course of getting sick and still be contagious. I stayed in a nearby hotel and limited my exposure to my son and his family. I kept socially distant and wore my N95 mask. They wore their own version of face coverings.

I didn't want my family to get sick, but I must have been doing a good job protecting myself as much as I was surrounded by the virus. We decided as a family to do all we could reasonably with being physically apart and wearing masks, but also needed to take time to visit and catch up. I didn't get the opportunity to see them much, so it was important. But so was keeping them safe. What a mental and emotional dilemma. It kept me up at night. I so desperately wanted to see my first grandbaby, and at the same time, was afraid to get near her.

The CDC recommends ten to fourteen-day quarantining after any exposure to people sick with COVID. Healthcare workers are swimming in coronavirus muck and we are protecting ourselves as much as possible with the PPE provided by the hospitals. This reduces our exposure risk, but not to zero. It is essentially impossible to quarantine from one's family with daily COVID exposure. Many nurses and doctors who I work with are sleeping in separate rooms from their spouses, wearing masks inside their homes, and maintaining social distancing as much as they can. Some are still getting sick.

Early on in this crisis, the Governor of New York recognized this to be a problem. I saw on the news that on March 25, he instituted a program in conjunction with Ty Warner Hotels and Resorts, allowing healthcare workers responding to the outbreak access to a hotel room free of charge to be able to protect their families by living apart. Many healthcare workers were already paying to stay at a hotel to keep their loved ones safe. Now they could feel supported by the city of New York. It tremendously helped boost morale of the healthcare workers in that state. I hope more cities and states will unite in helping healthcare workers keep their families protected with this example.

August 31, 2020

	COVID CASES		COVID DEATHS	
JAN	Global 12,308	US 1	Global 265	US 0
FEB	Global 86,471	US 60	Global 2,978	US 0
MAR	Global 889,005	US 149,378	Global 45,236	US 5,210
APR	Global 3,482,232	US 1,086,625	Global 238,993	US 62,955
MAY	Global 6,515,313	US 1,856,560	Global 382,743	US 108,439
JUN	Global 10,575,194	US 2,762,809	Global 526,357	US 129,710
JUL	Global 17,627,792	US 4,708,945	Global 694,078	US 157,386
AUG	Global 26,012,690	US 6,234,482	Global 866,636	US 187,596

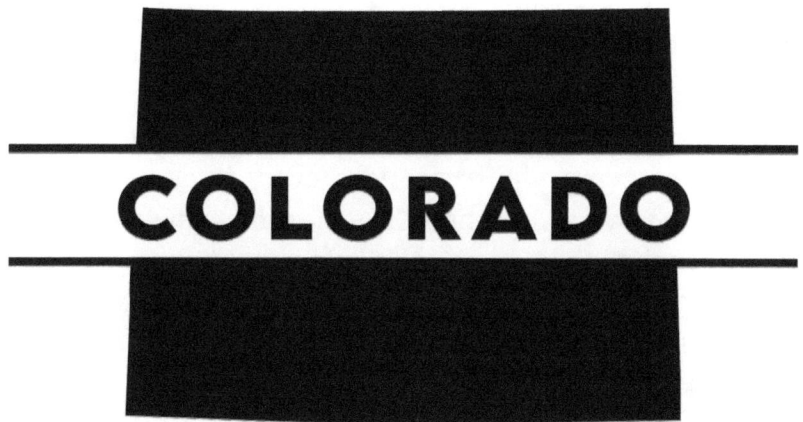

September 1, 2020

I left Tampa early to arrive home just in time to surprise my wife for her birthday. I tried to forget my time in Miami as I drove. It was hard to do. Images of those super sick patients in that swirling non-stop confusion with no relief in sight kept popping into my mind. The deaths were so high there. In my experience in Miami, only one lady out of all my ICU patients made it out alive.

Every year Sandra tells us she is celebrating the X (insert a random number here) anniversary of her 39th birthday. Even after cancer, she still looks much younger than anyone her age. As a cancer patient, Sandra is more at risk for serious complications if she gets this horrible disease. With her decreased immunity from this malignancy and the ongoing chemo treatments she has to take every three weeks, she cannot fight virus infections like healthy individuals. She already deals with so much and thinks about her mortality on a constant basis. Sandra says it would be a shame to survive cancer just to die from COVID. It's not going to happen to her—not if I can help it.

This pandemic is a big stressor in Sandra's life. When she goes to the grocery store, she wonders if the person near her in the check-out line has coronavirus. She has to be sequestered at home and can't do her usual social activities. And my love is home alone when I'm away working. I can't wrap her in my arms to comfort her when she is feeling bad after a treatment or when she gets scared if she's going to die from cancer or from COVID.

When I arrived, while I wanted to hug her so badly, we did what was safest. We kept socially distant and wore N95 masks. I stayed in a guest bedroom on another level at home for the recommended fourteen-day quarantine period. To finally be home with my wife was wonderful. But then to stay physically separated when she was right there was painful.

When I work, I work hard, but when I play, I play really hard. We filled our time with routine house maintenance chores and outdoor play activities. Elise and Logan both took their motorcycle safety class while I was away and have their permits to ride. Riding in a group is a lot of fun, especially if it is all your family.

Sandra and I took the kids on their maiden voyage through Evergreen to a touristy coffee shop. Short rides are best for these young riders to get experience and confidence. They need to get more exposure to taking tight curves like switchbacks and learning how to handle steep inclines. I'm grateful to be able to help them become better and safer riders.

September 3, 2020

I'm feeling like I am starting to become human again. Communication is much different with my wife at home than at work with my co-workers or vented patients who are sedated that I am with all day long. Here I get all the little questions like "How are you feeling today? How did you sleep? What would you like to eat for supper tonight? Which trail would you like to take?" I forget how I miss that attention.

At work I'm on a runner's high all the time, ramped up on adrenaline. I can understand how it is easy to get addicted to that energized feeling. Here at home, my emotions are upside down, high and low. Don't get me wrong, I love my wife and love being home. It just takes time to transition from being 'GO, GO, GO' all the time to calm down to normal life. It is like a car on a racetrack going two hundred miles per hour versus taking a Sunday drive with the top down on back roads at a leisurely pace.

Getting out in nature with Sandra helps me restore quickly. There is enough open space to be able to keep socially distant on a trail, even if someone isn't wearing the mandated mask. Summer and fall activities are great in Colorado, but they are not the only season I enjoy. As a Black man who grew up in the South, most think I cannot tolerate cold and would not be found dead on skis or a snowboard. Snowboarding is one of my favorite winter sports. I am optimistic that COVID will soon be conquered, and we will be able to safely get back to the slopes again—in a year or two.

September 7, 2020

I have been riding bikes for years and have had the pleasure to go to the huge motorcycle rally in Sturgis, South Dakota twice. It was lots of fun, but very dangerous because of the many attitudes that come with bikers.

There are the One Percenters, the tough guys. These are the men and women who really give the image or stereotype of bad asses. And they really are bad asses! They are in motorcycle clubs or MCs, which have repercussions, if you don't follow all the rules. I heard that in several gangs, you have to sign your bike over to the club. If you decide to get out, you have to leave your bike behind. Initiation into some gangs can involve illegal activity like breaking into a store or house, stealing valuables, and even possibly killing someone. Of course, I can't confirm any of this at all. I know my place in the motorcycle riding world. The majority of bikers who want to stay out of trouble belong to Riding Groups. You won't get beat up if you forget to do something right. They just enjoy riding for the sake of riding.

The rally at Sturgis usually has about 500,000 attending every year. Most bikers are put in the category of being rebels. Breaking coronavirus rules was no exception. There was a slight drop from normal with 450,000 people there this year, but there shouldn't have been any at all. The smart ones want to live to ride another day and not catch the Rona and possibly die or kill their family.

Two weeks later guess what happened? That's right, another coronavirus explosion. Cases blew up in the Dakotas, Montana, Wyoming, and Minnesota. Do people realize that there is a virus spreading across the entire planet killing people?

September 8, 2020

Even though we stay busy doing fun activities, it is always in the back of my mind I will be leaving soon. I looked at the assignment list many times daily, much to my wife's dismay. She tried to get me to not open those emails. The pull is hard because every day there are hundreds of available nursing positions across the US for ICU and ED nurses. The areas hardest hit at this time seem to be southern California, Texas, and Arizona. In all my professional travels, I usually end up in a big urban area in big city hospitals.

There was a posting for a small rural hospital close to Bakersfield, California that was catching my eye. I had worked in rural Colorado before and know these hospitals suffered the most. They usually only have twenty-five beds or less and finances are always tight. Maybe I should try a change of pace this time. The wildfires in California were out of control this year. Even right now there were some campers who are trapped. Should I really go from the COVID frying pan into a real California fire?

My wife is a Chief Medical Officer of a physician's group that serves mostly rural hospitals throughout the country. She is always talking about how medicine in the rural community is personal and rewarding. In a big city, a hospital has thousands of employees and nobody knows anyone. There is no time to spend getting to know your patients, much less the co-workers.

She tells me how patients who come to the hospital in a small town are the neighbors or family members of someone working in the hospital. Nobody is a stranger. After orientation, a traveler is usually taken around to each department in the facility and introduced to feel at home. The word gets around that a new nurse is there. It's that hometown warm welcome I will love. Small Town, USA, here I come!

September 15, 2020

The news had many reports about the dire situation in southern California. Hospitals were begging for nurses more and more every day. Several of the small hospitals that partner with Sandra's company related they were unable to staff their units adequately for the patients who were coming in the door. Large hospitals on the west coast were full and struggling in the same way. I had only been home less than three weeks and didn't feel recharged yet. Just thinking of leaving my love so soon brought tears to my eyes. I had to take many deep breaths over the last few days. Sandra noticed and asked me what I was doing. I said that just the thought of leaving her hurt my soul. But if I went now, I could get home in time for Christmas.

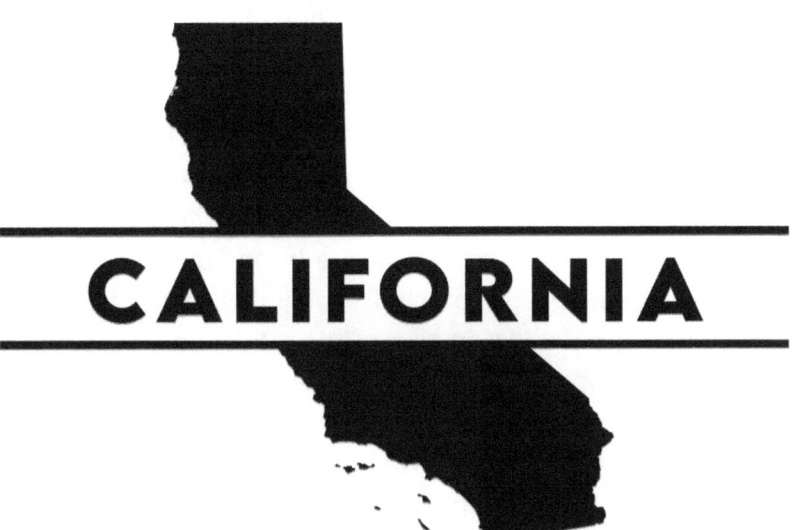

September 19, 2020

I drove mainly in silence, contemplating what I might encounter in this new hospital. Already I was missing Sandra and the comfort of home. It wasn't just the home cooked meals or the outside activities—her companionship is what I miss the most. We talk a lot on the phone when I'm gone and yet, I can't caress her cheek or cradle her in my arms while I sleep. I just don't feel whole without her. It sounds really cliché or corny and that's the truth of my feelings for my wife.

Driving to southern California was so beautiful it distracted me from my sadness. The route from interstate 70 to 15 to 58—divine! I had to take many photos of the changing rocks on the mountains. Not subtle changes, but dramatic changes in the giants towering over me as I drove through canyons and valleys. Colors of grays, blues, reds, and purples bounced off the massive pieces of land protruding from the earth, reaching to the sky like fingers of the tallest person reaching for the sun. I was unsure if I was chasing the light of day or driving away from darkness as I saw the night catching up to me through my rearview mirror. I finally made it into this gem of a town called Tehachapi.

September 22, 2020

After being here for a few days, I came to realize that a lot of the residents never have been anywhere else in the US. This is common for most regular folks. Traveling isn't always on the minds of hardworking citizens because it is expensive, and they can't afford to take time off work.

I am lucky to be able to travel with my job. It allows me to go to places that have been stuck away and hidden from the rest of the world, a lot like this little town. This area is like having a slice of God's apple pie and a latte made by Mother Nature. Folks here really have no desire for an influx of people moving in on their sacred land. I hear gossip of big companies buying up property, building big businesses and housing communities in the near future. I think this is a very good thing for the economy here, but I wouldn't want it to lose its small-town charm.

Big businesses in the area will also stimulate growth of local healthcare. This town comes with a hospital that was quickly becoming one of my favorite places to work. The folks here have been the most amazing group of people I have ever worked with throughout my career. My first encounter was an interview with the ICU manager, Angela. Even though she is busy and wears many hats at work, she spends time with her nurses, which shows how special she is as a leader. She is kind and cares for each and every one of us. Angela and all my other co-workers accepted me not just as an employee, but they made me feel like I was part of a family. I felt like a big brother coming home from a war after being away for a long time. From Day One they treated me like I was someone special and not just another warm body to put on the schedule. The entire community is the same. It's like a real-life town of Mayberry from the *Andy Griffith Show*.

Tehachapi General is part of a faith-based hospital system. Every morning and evening, the nurses meet in the break room to receive their assignments. It shocked me when we all held hands and prayed the first time I went to the break room to start our day. I have never in my twenty plus years said a prayer before going out on the floors in a hospital. This was not just a one-day thing; this was every single workday. I have to admit whether you are religious or not, to pray, or meditate, or come together as a group puts you in a different frame of mind. It helps keep focus on the patients and the bigger picture, rather than personal problems. It also helps us nurses feel like we are a team instead of being out there alone taking care of the sick. I definitely feel an inner strength after our prayers.

September 23, 2020

My gig is a long thirteen-week assignment. Whenever I've started a new deployment during this crisis, it usually is pandemonium, with emergencies constantly being called overhead and hospital employees running around trying to do their jobs. I was expecting this town of 13,000 people to be overrun with COVID throughout the hospital and the community.

It was surprising to discover an almost empty hospital. There were only three patients admitted and five additional patients getting short-term rehabilitation. That was it. Where are all the sick patients? Does COVID not exist in this town in southern California? In the six months since the outbreak began, they have only seen eighty positive COVID admissions and had twenty coronavirus deaths. These are miniscule numbers compared to big city urban areas. Why did they need me?

I quickly discovered some challenges unique to a small town. Most of the nurses live locally and there are not many of them. When these nurses get sick, there is no one to pick up the slack. Fill-in travelers usually prefer to go to larger cities to have more options for things to do on their days off. They rarely accept assignments in rural towns. There was a surge of COVID admissions just before I arrived and the nurses here are not wanting to face that again without help.

Some of the doctors working here also work in Los Angeles. They fully understand the tide that is coming this way again, probably in a few weeks. The media is predicting that hospitals in large metropolitan areas will quickly run out of beds. They will not be able to help us if we needed to transfer a critically ill patient requiring a higher level of care. Those patients would have to stay here regardless of how sick they become. We would have to care for everyone who comes in the door. Those big urban hospitals will be calling us to take their overflow patients who are being held in the emergency room for days waiting for an empty bed. I am starting to feel a little anxiety as to what is likely to hit this small town. The nurses here will soon be overrun with more patients than they have ever seen in their entire careers. How will we all manage?

September 24, 2020

Today, I had one ICU patient who only spoke Spanish which made communication very difficult. (I see with this pandemic I need to learn español.) He was on a BiPAP machine, which made speaking impossible anyway. His family wanted to video chat with him, but he could not be without his mask for less than a minute before becoming incoherent. Every time he took his mask off to swallow medications, his oxygen dropped dangerously into the 70s and his lips turned blue. He became anxious and short of breath. This poor guy was scared out of his mind, like all my patients at this stage. I had seen this so many times before, I knew what was coming. He would quickly need more breathing support and would get the tube. The rest of this day was spent with us struggling to get his oxygen up to at least 90% to sustain his life.

September 25, 2020

I was reassigned to the ICU. The man from yesterday was my patient again. I got in report that he made it through the night and was still on BiPAP. The patient needed his morning meds, so I went through the entire process of gathering the things needed to enter a COVID room and put on all the PPE.

 As I entered the room, my patient stared up at me with tremendous fear of impending doom. His eyes rolled back, his face turned blue, his heart rate dropped to 35, then he lost his pulse. I immediately jumped to hit the code blue button on the wall. After checking again for a pulse and not finding one, I started compressions. The room instantly became filled with staff to try to resuscitate him. After thirty-five minutes of CPR, his pulse miraculously returned. We added medications that would hopefully keep him stable. I took this opportunity to call his family to notify them about what happened.

We as healthcare providers in COVID understand once a patient starts decompensating like this, we will likely go through code blue scenarios multiple times a day until the patient dies. In my experience, the ICU mortality in older patients or those with additional health problems is almost 100%. This patient was not likely to survive even with CPR and all our fancy medications and treatments for this coronavirus.

The physician and I discussed with the family that the situation was grim. The likelihood of their loved one surviving this critical COVID ordeal is very low. We asked if they would consider end of life comfort measures only. It is very hard to let go, which is understandable. No one wants to say goodbye to their loved one. Every hospital has people to support and guide you with making the best decisions for you and your family. But ultimately, those decisions are very personal choices. Comfort measures is when we would do everything to keep the patient without pain or suffering, but with the understanding death was imminent. CPR or other life-saving measures would not be implemented.

CPR is brutal. Breaking ribs is unavoidable as the pressure we use pushing on the chest is intended to compress the heart mimicking a heartbeat. Ribs cannot withstand that type of compressive force at 100 beats per minute. If we continue the code for 30 minutes, that is 3,000 compressions. We have to push in the chest 2 ½ inches to reach the heart and circulate blood. That is what pops those ribs. They don't bend.

The patient's family had strong religious beliefs that prohibit giving up, even in hopeless situations. The Latino community is generally very religious, and many are Catholic. As I understand it, Catholics believe if you do not actively try to save a person with everything possible it is a sin. Pulling the plug is not acceptable. I understand the anguish the family must have been feeling, torn between their religious beliefs and not wanting to cause more pain and suffering.

We in the medical community feel that when the situation is hopeless, we wish to provide the patient comfort for a painless death. He ended up today with many fractured ribs and both lungs ruptured from the CPR we performed. I was busy with him all day long and couldn't leave his room even for lunch. We coded him at 8 a.m. and thirteen times more before he finally passed away at 5:43 p.m. This poor man went through unbearable torture each and every code. It didn't save him in the long run.

This is the usual routine in an ICU with COVID patients. It is utterly horrible. I have seen more death in these six months than I have seen in my whole entire life. There is no good way to die, but the ways of death with this infection are the worst.

During a code, every two minutes we are giving meds and doing CPR, giving more meds and doing CPR, shocking the patient and doing CPR, on, and on, and on. Every time a medication is administered, titrated, or changed, we will eventually need to document this in the patient's chart.

In most hospitals, IV pumps interface with the computer system. In an emergency like the one we had today where multiple medications were started and doses changed numerous times in an hour, it is automatically documented. I was constantly titrating drugs all day long and didn't even think to write this down manually. My supervisor came to me at the end of my shift and told me that before I went home, I had to think back and document every single time I adjusted the drips responding to the patient's changing condition to document the exact time it was done—oh yeah, right!

Their electronic medical record system is actually sophisticated enough to automatically document, but they didn't have it set up yet. I wonder what it will be like here when we have patients in every room and lining the hallways. When the coronavirus apocalypse comes to life in this neck of the woods, we will need efficiencies like IV pump/computer interfaces to make our day manageable.

September 26, 2020

Being so welcome here made me think back to my first day in New Jersey when I also felt at home. Most of my career, I have worked at many hospitals and have been the only Black nurse. I'm sure it has a lot to do with the demographics of the region. I was excited to not only see Black nurses in New Jersey, but three or four Black male nurses! Those are a rare breed indeed. Can you imagine how it must feel as a Black man from the South to be the only Black nurse in an entire hospital? How do you think a White nurse would feel if they had to work in a hospital with an entirely Black staff? Wouldn't it feel weird? Well, I don't feel weird here even though I am in the minority.

On my one or two days off each week, I went on long hikes in the beautiful mountains to reset my spirit. I filled my phone full of photos of huge trees and gorgeous trails. Driving on those roads with the steep switch backs, twisting every which way with thousand-foot cliffs only a foot away was terrifying, but fun!

I took the opportunity being out here in Cali to go see the Sequoias. When I saw the forest of gargantuan trees thousands of years old, I thought about how many people and animals have actually lived to see this amazing gift from the heavens. When I took in this scenery straight from a medieval fairy tale, I knew there had to be a God. The biggest and oldest tree was called the General. When I laid eyes on that monster, I thought of exactly that—prehistoric monsters like T-Rex! I wonder what it must have been like in that time in history. No grocery stores to get food, no hospitals to get care, no cars for transportation, no computers, no internet, but it sure was beautiful.

September 28, 2020

In the beginning of the outbreak in New Jersey and New York, I was the only one wearing an N95. Everyone else wore surgical masks at first. Healthcare workers dropped like flies, and I am still without any sign of the virus. So far in this hospital, nobody is wearing N95 masks unless they go into a COVID-positive room. The same thing will happen like in New Jersey and New York. Nurses will get sick quickly if they don't start protecting themselves.

    This must be the reason they needed me. Hospital administration must be anticipating another surge. I hope they also see examples in other states and raise the level of protection requirements for their employees soon. I know I will continue to wear my N95 everywhere I go and always add a PAPR (if it is available) with my N95 when I care for COVID patients.

Sept 30, 2020

	COVID CASES		COVID DEATHS	
JAN	Global 12,308	US 1	Global 265	US 0
FEB	Global 86,471	US 60	Global 2,978	US 0
MAR	Global 889,005	US 149,378	Global 45,236	US 5,210
APR	Global 3,482,232	US 1,086,625	Global 238,993	US 62,955
MAY	Global 6,515,313	US 1,856,560	Global 382,743	US 108,439
JUN	Global 10,575,194	US 2,762,809	Global 526,357	US 129,710
JUL	Global 17,627,792	US 4,708,945	Global 694,078	US 157,386
AUG	Global 26,012,690	US 6,234,482	Global 866,636	US 187,596
SEP	Global 34,891,132	US 7,532,411	Global 1,020,526	US 212,082

October 5, 2020

I smell smoke all the time. It's all around me. Just like I've seen the red glow of the wildfires burning since August. I read a lot on the internet about these wildfires in California that have burned almost four million acres so far this year. To put this in perspective, the worst year in California history was 2018 when around 1.8 million acres burned. This is now more than double and it's still going. Over 50,000 people are displaced from their homes so far. What is this doing to the wildlife? Where will they go to escape? It's incredible to think of yet another additional level of suffering happening this year. The sun reflecting off the ash in the air helps create vivid sunrises and sunsets. That at least is one tiny consolation to all the displacement and loss that is occurring in these California rural communities and along the West coast.

October 9, 2020

It was like any other day to me except our low patient census. We had four patients on the Medical Surgical Unit and two patients in the ICU. I was assigned to work on the Med Surg side. Under normal circumstances, I would expect an easy peaceful day with two nurses taking care of two patients each and three of them were going home. But that was not what happened.

I was sitting at the nurse's station charting on my two patients when I heard a loud deep male voice booming, "You fuckin' bitch, get outta my room! You hurt my leg!"

I ran to see what the commotion was about. This patient was a fifty-year-old male admitted to the hospital for an infected leg. This man was about 6'6" and 260 pounds; that was a big man. As I entered the room, I noticed his extremely swollen leg hanging partway off the bed with multiple open wounds. It was all related to shooting up crack and other hard drugs to get him that next high. He had a raging MRSA infection in his leg. His nurse tried to get him set up for his daily care routine as he would do on his own. He insisted that she give him a shower. She refused since this grown man was highly capable of showering himself.

He turned toward me and yelled, "She is a muthafuckin' bitch! She hurt my leg, and I don't want her touchin' me again. They treat me like this just because I'm Black. They haven't treated me right since I been here."

I stared at him, unable to come up with words. I was in shock he could say this about this sweet lady nurse. She wears skirts and dresses for her uniform, which I haven't seen since I worked in a Catholic hospital with nuns. The patient looked at me and said with a tone in his voice like I would automatically agree with him, "Bro, you know how they treat us. It ain't right, my nigga."

I responded, "I am a Black American man as well as you, and I've never had anyone in this hospital discriminate against me or any other Black patient. Please refrain from cussing at our staff and cooperate. Be nice to her. She is one of the best nurses here." The patient seemed to listen to what I said and actually calmed down—for a short minute.

The lady nurse went to get the shower prepared for him and left to take care of her other patients. When he got up on his own two feet, I saw this adult man had crapped in his bed. I can't believe a person in their right mind would even consider doing such a thing. Grabbing a fresh sheet, I cleaned it up, so the sweet lady nurse didn't have to endure any more from this man.

He made many wrong decisions, including the one to bad mouth and berate this nice nurse; the sweetest, most caring of all the nurses in this hospital. This lady honestly always goes above and beyond to give more than what her patients need.

When I returned to the nurses' station, I called the physician and explained about the unsafe environment the inappropriate, aggressive patient was causing. The doc reviewed the patient's case and decided it was safe to discharge him to a shelter closer to his relatives and prescribed oral antibiotics for his infection. The patient tried to convince the doc to let him stay. I'm sure it was because he had a warm bed and three square meals a day. The doc did not back down, and the patient finally accepted his discharge orders.

We called for a cab. As the patient waited, the door to his room was wide open. He was loudly speaking on the phone. It sounded like he was using code to talk about something illegal and it seemed like he owed someone a lot of money. I did not want to get into all of that, but paid attention just in case he threatened my co-workers again.

It was about 4 p.m. when he walked to the nurses' station and leaned over the counter towards the sweet lady nurse. "Where's that fuckin' doctor? He said he would give me a Motrin prescription for my pain. He's probably takin' a shit somewhere and ignorin' me, like all y'all White folks." The staff around the sweet lady nurse responded in respectful tones, trying to help him understand that the doctor was in the ED admitting other patients and that Motrin was inexpensive and available over the counter without a prescription. It seemed to me they were bending over backwards to help this guy despite his abusive language and hostile behavior.

I have never worked in a hospital where the staff spoil the patients to the level they do here. These hospital employees treat patients like royalty. They even paid for his cab fare. I'm sure he knew he was going to a harsher place.

We made eye contact and he said to me, "Bro, you know what I mean. They don't care about us. This is some bullshit."

I said, "Sir, this is a Christian hospital, and we have patients in the other rooms that can hear everything you're saying. You will not use vulgar language anymore."

He approached me and got in my face. "Fuck you, nigga. We can go right now."

I pointed to the doors and I said, "Go, get out of this hospital. You have made too many threats and we have given you too many chances. GET OUT NOW, SIR!" Turning to the nurse I said, "Call Security. STAT!"

As I escorted him down the hall, he said, "You just a fuckin' Oreo."

"They go good with milk. Have a blessed day and be safe out there," I responded. There was no point in me taking his verbal abuse as a personal attack. I didn't understand how enforcing peace in the workplace could be misconstrued as me being a 'yes man' for White people.

He said, "If I wasn't on parole, I would take care of you, nigga."

I remained professional and replied, "We tried to help you and take care of you. Make sure to get your antibiotics or your leg will get worse."

This incident reminded me of the Neo Nazi patient I took care of who had numerous swastika tattoos. Even though he obviously had racist views, the man spoke to me with respect, and we had normal everyday conversations. I did not feel discriminated against by that patient at any time I cared for him. Not like this Black guy today. How bizarre that even Black folks can be racist to other Black folks. How is that even possible?

I asked the House Supervisor to make sure the patient got in the taxi and drove away. He was the type of person who would wait for any of us to come outside, then retaliate. I have known health care workers who were followed home by disgruntled patients or even murdered outside of a hospital. That did not happen today.

October 21, 2020

Since I was just in Miami, the headline this morning caught my eye. They were having king tides in addition to heavy rain. A few times a year the full moon decides to do a greater gravitational pull when it is closest to the sun, creating these larger than normal tides. It's like soaking in a full bathtub and then your song comes on and you start movin' to the groovin', water splashing everywhere. I felt sorry for the healthcare workers having to go back and forth from their homes to work trying to drive through that.

It's still hurricane season. This storm should have been named because it was so big, but it was not classified as an official hurricane. Besides, all the names are taken. They have already gone through the entire regular alphabet and they had to bust out the fricking Greek alphabet in mid-September with two months left to go. Epsilon is around Bermuda and bringing more king tides to the east coast. When they go through to Omega, will they use Cyrillic, or maybe Kanji next?

October 22, 2020

I saw on the internet the FDA announced remdesivir to be the first antiviral medicine approved to treat COVID, but only for hospitalized patients. The studies proved it shortened patients' course in the hospital. That's great progress in such a short time. Thousands of scientists are racing to find safe solutions wherever they are in the world.

With case numbers rising by the minute, people were rushing out to grab onto any Holy Grail they can find. A news article discussed how many Latin American countries were using Ivermectin as a treatment for COVID. This presents several problems. Originally, it was used for livestock to treat things like parasitic worms and then it was developed for human use. Clinical trials are difficult to do because so many people are getting it through different means. Since the human grade medicine is in short supply, people are using the animal version on the black market. This is unsafe in every which way. I also read about a small study they conducted in Israel in June but it needed more patients to be scientifically significant. There may be some merit in this medicine, but only time and larger safe clinical trials will tell.

October 29, 2020

Looking back on that first day with the tall Korean man, I had no idea of the tsunami about to slam into all of our lives. During this COVID year, a lot was done well, and a great many things were a complete failure.

The Governor of New York shut the Big Apple down early in this crisis when it became the epicenter. I was right there in the middle of it. He put the whole state on a full lockdown in March and April. There were no big events like weddings or concerts or political rallies. There was a limit of only ten to twenty folks maximum at any gathering and a $15,000 fine if you chose to hold the event anyway. There were restrictions for restaurants, bars, and gyms to close at 10 p.m., but take-out didn't have a time limitation. There was even a social distancing fine of $1,000. Testing was free to New Yorkers. And of course, they tracked and isolated all the positive people. I saw this city actually turn around and patients started surviving. By the summer, New York had less than 1% new cases per day and never did see the "summer second wave," like many other states. Even today, New York is not half as bad as other areas in the United States. Those early tough restrictions seemed to make a big difference in that overpopulated region of our country.

Some countries around the world got ahold of this crisis fast. It made a huge difference in places like New Zealand and Australia, among many others. There were a lot of reports looking at their strategies, and how they closed their borders quickly and did not allow mass gatherings like political rallies and other large events. They allowed testing to be free and encouraged everyone feeling sick to get tested. Of course, they also tracked and isolated COVID-positive patients immediately.

One remarkable difference I read about was that citizens in other countries have been supportive of their government's mandated guidelines and regulations. Those citizens viewed these changes that impacted their individual personal rights as necessary to save the lives of their fellow countrymen. It is like the 1-2 knockout punch in a fight with COVID… which end of the glove do you want to be on when it is a matter of life and death?

October 31, 2020

It was Halloween, but I had been dressed in a space suit most days since March. I am so tired of the elevated PPE requirements. It would be great if we could go back to the way it was before. This year seems like one long horror movie morphing into the next with monster hurricanes or racial conflicts or colossal wildfires or political conspiracies. Seeing my patients today brought me flashbacks of the busier hospitals overflowing with suffering patients. I remembered the rooms being double occupancy with every patient on a ventilator, with even more patients stationed in the hallway labeled as "Room 206C." I feel physical chest pain and claustrophobic just thinking about those days earlier in this fight. There are no adequate words to describe the insanity. I keep repeating how it's like a war. It's the only description that can come close to this nightmare. Those who have been in battle, I hope you can understand this comparison.

	COVID CASES		COVID DEATHS	
JAN	Global 12,308	US 1	Global 265	US 0
FEB	Global 86,471	US 60	Global 2,978	US 0
MAR	Global 889,005	US 149,378	Global 45,236	US 5,210
APR	Global 3,482,232	US 1,086,625	Global 238,993	US 62,955
MAY	Global 6,515,313	US 1,856,560	Global 382,743	US 108,439
JUN	Global 10,575,194	US 2,762,809	Global 526,357	US 129,710
JUL	Global 17,627,792	US 4,708,945	Global 694,078	US 157,386
AUG	Global 26,012,690	US 6,234,482	Global 866,636	US 187,596
SEP	Global 34,891,132	US 7,532,411	Global 1,020,526	US 212,082
OCT	Global 47,161,108	US 9,395,274	Global 1,202,691	US 235,492

November 3, 2020

Even though I was taking care of patients, I was able to watch the election count. It was almost impossible to avoid because it was on every TV in the hospital. America was divided and people were completely polarized. Even though traditionally I do not identify with either side of our political arena, I hope for a kind and more peaceful leadership. On top of the pandemic, I feel like I am in between a political and racial war. It's hard enough to deal with just one of these issues, much less all three at once. I guess that was what has pushed many to cast their votes.

This was an extraordinary event. So many people voted! The media said it was the largest turnout in any election since President William McKinley won in 1900. Many voted by mail to remain safe sheltering at home. Others waited in long lines to vote at their appointed stations. Due to social distancing regulations, the lines stretched out the doors into the cold winter weather. Many celebrities and public figures made appeals during the last few months encouraging people to cast their ballots. It worked. Over 150 million Americans voted, including more than 55% of eligible young people. It was great to see our youth take such an interest in issues shaping our nation. They have made many stands this year and I hope they are going to be good leaders in our future.

Waiting for the count is difficult. The polls are extremely close in several states leading to many ballot recounts. Let's see how long this will take; probably days. I'll be holding my breath with suspense and I'm sure everyone else is too.

November 6, 2020

It's been a very tough year for millions of families across the globe. I never thought I would hear, "We have no more body bags." The first sensation I felt when I heard that phrase was how surreal and eerie that sounded. Then I shuddered with the reality of it. Etched in my brain is that all those corpses in more than a quarter of a million body bags across the entire US were alive last year and none of them anticipated this outcome. And worst of all, I have heard this terrifying phrase in every single hospital I've worked in since March.

Here in rural southern California, it's been relatively calm so far. We've had some cases, but it's not anything like the urban cities. Two hours away, Los Angeles is getting hit hard and I anticipate it will be here soon. Part of me feels like I need to be in LA and part of me is happy to have this little break. Not just from the overwhelming work every single minute, but from the war-like horror that doesn't end. Even when I was at home, I couldn't stop thinking about my patients and their immense suffering, along with their families' grief. It was horrible.

In my experience, I saw how this disease took lives, but also broke up families and relationships. I read how domestic violence and child abuse was on the rise. The foster care system was hit hard with children needing placement. But fewer people qualified with many layoffs across the country. This is America, supposedly the top nation in the entire world. It sure doesn't feel like it anymore. Will we ever go back to the way life used to be before?

In the beginning of this nightmare, New York City was the epicenter of the pandemic in the US with hundreds of deaths every day. I know because I was there. It was not logical to think that every single one of those unfortunate souls had a next of kin. There were several articles online talking about how more than 650 bodies in New York still to this day are waiting in freezers. Their relatives could not be found. Few people carry a card in their wallet saying, "Please notify so and so if I am incapacitated." Most probably arrived in the ER with shortness of breath. Then they died quickly and were put in one of those body bags. Many were not registered in the hospital and there was no contact information. We really do our best to let next of kin know what happened. But what do we do when we don't have that vital information? I have also seen entire families dying. Who do you call then? That just does not even seem like it could be real.

November 7, 2020

The count and wait was over. The winner is President-Elect Joe Biden. Trump claimed the election was stolen and fraudulent with all kinds of lawsuits in the works. I wonder what will happen if this is not resolved by the time Congress formally counts the electoral votes on January 6. What will happen on Inauguration Day on the 20th?

Regardless of who you voted for, Kamala Harris is most notable in this election securing three firsts in history. She is the first woman Vice President, the first Asian American Vice President, and the first Black American Vice President. Congratulations to her!

November 13, 2020

Finally, the fires are out. California coined a term—gigafire. It's a rare designation for a blaze that burns a million acres or more. I'm looking forward to clearer skies and breathing easier. Especially I hope there won't be cause to use that word again. All of us have disaster fatigue, COVID fatigue, discrimination fatigue, domestic violence fatigue, police brutality fatigue, wildfire fatigue, political division fatigue, hurricane fatigue, etc... I know I do. It's exhausting.

Hurricane season is finally over, and it was unprecedented. The record shows thirty storms, thirteen hurricanes, twelve made land fall, and six were major. It's so mind boggling, I tend to forget all the details of the other unbelievable unprecedented amounts of other unprecedented events.

November 14, 2020

Today was Saturday and I was assigned to the emergency room. My day started off sitting with a young psychiatric patient in his early twenties who was suicidal. He seemed like a nice enough guy but he was not seeing life clearly. It makes me sad to see many young folks trying to end their lives before they even really started living.

There were paramedic students here to get clinical hours from time to time and we always appreciate their tremendous help. I caught a glimpse in my peripheral view of one of the students walking past my patient's room. A brief second later, I saw someone hurrying behind him, so I turned my head to get a better look. It was another psychiatric patient who had just checked in to the emergency department. He followed the student to the corner room and started throwing punches out of nowhere. I saw the first punch thrown as the student ducked. The student tried to take the patient down. The patient threw a second punch and clocked the student in the back of the head. In my mind, everything slowed down to real s-l-o-w motion, like the *Six Million Dollar Man*, Lee Majors, slow motion.

I fought MMA for five years and trained four to six hours a day consistently. It was my life. There was nothing like when I stepped into the cage knowing I was prepared to whoop ass no matter what on fight night. My trainers and coaches had me psyched up. I could feel the heat of the big lights overhead in the cage beaming down on my skin, the crowd screaming my name, and my fight song booming on the PA system. That adrenaline is like primordial wild dinosaur kind of adrenaline. Well, I had flashbacks of my MMA days, and instantly went into motion.

I ran to stop the patient who was violently assaulting the unsuspecting student. As he came around with a right elbow at my head, I jammed his swing, and placed him in a rear naked choke. Then we went to the mat—or the tile floor, in this case. As soon as we hit the floor, my arm kept his face from connecting hard on the ground and he started tapping. I whispered in his ear, "This is not an MMA fight. You can't tap out. You assaulted a student for no reason."

He yelled, "I give up!"

I kept whispering, "We are here to help you and you do this?!"

He gasped. "I can't breathe."

As I kept my chokehold on him, I started thinking about George Floyd. There was no way I was going to kill this punk, and I loosened my grip just enough to let him breathe, but not so he could get loose. I was still in the zone when the ED Charge Nurse placed her hand on my shoulder and spoke softly in a motherly tone, "Nico, it is okay. You can let him go now." I released my grip when more help arrived.

It took a couple of hours for my rush to go away. I felt like I was flying with nervous energy and excitement, just like when I finished a battle in the cage. A little while later, I started feeling my old fight injury in my knee. I'm much more of a lover than a fighter nowadays. Yet, if anyone tries to beat up staff in any hospital I'm working in at any time, I'm definitely up to schooling those young bucks in the art of appropriate conduct in a hospital.

November 17, 2020

I read today about how oil prices dropped back in April. The suppliers ran out of storage room and had to pay distributors to store the excess oil, making the official price negative $30 a barrel. In the entire history of the oil industry, this number has never gone below zero. A decrease in oil prices would mean a drop in fuel prices, which would have a domino effect on our economy. Supply and demand. However, since we are in a pandemic, nobody should be going anywhere anyway.

On the other hand, the mental stressors of being on lockdown are real. As an essential worker I don't personally feel the stress of a continued lockdown, but Sandra does. She tells me how stir-crazy she feels and how sometimes she just stands outside our front door to get a break from the closed walls of our house. Other people have it worse. Some in big cities live in apartments and do not have the fortune to be able to get outside away from others. Many children are home-schooling, so moms are the ones mostly having to decrease or stop their work. Dads might be working remotely from home and many have to tend to their children as well. Imagine being cooped up with your family for months and months on end. They have nowhere else to go during a stay-at-home order. This is causing a lot of depression and other mental health issues.

Even in some parts of healthcare, unemployment is up. Surgery centers had to lay off employees because elective surgeries were cancelled or indefinitely postponed. Other service businesses like restaurants and salons had to shut down, leaving people out of work. People can't pay their rent or mortgage, so homelessness is up despite a moratorium that landlords cannot evict. Domestic violence is at an all-time high. Suicide rates and divorce rates are also on the rise.

Is there a solution? As I sat with this guy on suicide watch, I was really sad about the younger generation having to suffer in this pandemic with all the new extreme stressors, and now many are feeling there is no way out. They haven't lived long enough to realize there is always another door. I do not have an answer for all this, but wish I could do more.

I was talking with a police chief when he came into the hospital the other day. I asked him, "How have you seen the pandemic affect the police force?"

He said, "I have to deal with many officers who are fighting with their spouses because all the overtime is taking them away from their families. One officer threatened all over social media to blow up his house with his wife in it. Now he's charged with a felony and labeled as a threat to society. It's so sad. We have to deal with many issues related to death threats and suicides on a frequent basis."

I answered, "We also are seeing higher than normal divorce rates and deaths among our ranks. But our deaths are not usually self-inflicted. How does it really feel to be a police officer these days? Lots of folks hate cops, does that make you feel uncomfortable?"

He said, "Absolutely. And we have to change this. Every time we make progress here locally, some idiot across the country pepper sprays a nine-year-old or shoots another Black jogger when he is out for his early morning run. Cops are necessary in our society, but that doesn't mean they can abuse their position."

Who would you call if someone was breaking into your house or trying to steal your car? The cops. Who would you call if someone was stalking you and you were afraid for your life? The cops. They are living in our community as our friends and neighbors. I wish the term peace officer would make a comeback. Most cops already live up to that name. Maybe one day our society will have a better opinion of our men in blue.

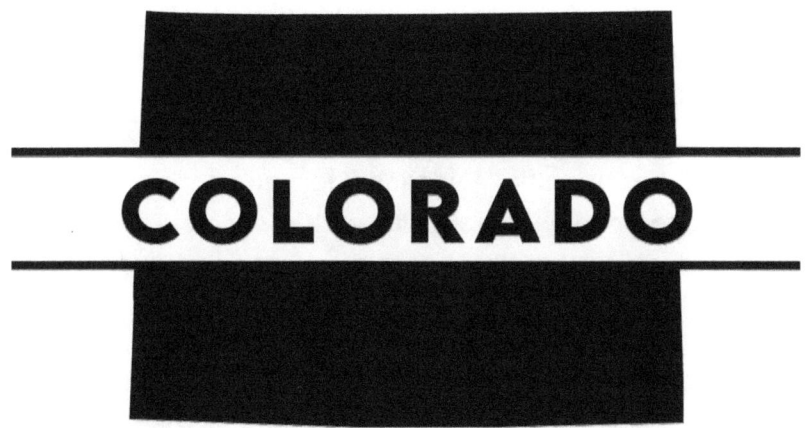

November 23, 2020

My assignment was not over yet, but I needed to see my wife for a few days for the Thanksgiving holiday. It would be our first one apart if I stayed here. I called Sandra.

"Hey baby, what's up?" Sandra asked.

"I've been gone for two months. I really want to see you. It is another four weeks before my assignment ends," I said.

Sandra answered. "I would love for you to come home, but there wouldn't be enough time to quarantine."

"I've been really, really careful. I've worn my N95 mask and another mask on top everywhere. I haven't had coronavirus this whole year. I should be safe," I explained.

"It's still a risk," she answered.

"I know baby, I know. But it's a low risk and it's Thanksgiving. The CDC has specific guidelines for quarantine after an exposure to people who are sick with the virus. I am always protected, so am I really in that group needing quarantine? I don't want you to be home alone for Thanksgiving." I said.

"I miss you, too. Is it worth the risk for only five days?" Sandra asked.

"I have taken extra precautions by wearing an N95 everywhere, even when I am off shift. When I see COVID patients, I wear the PAPR on top of the N95. I have tested numerous times and all tests have returned negative. I know I have been lucky. The N95 is not 100% effective, only 95%," I explained.

"Come home, baby, just come home," she answered.

"I love you. I'll make plans."

My heart was so happy I could feel it speeding up just visualizing my wife in my arms and smelling her beautiful hair. In order to spend as much time with Sandra as possible, I decided to get an airplane ticket to go home for the holidays.

Colorado

There's no way I will spend sixteen hours on the road, stay just three days, and turn around to drive all the way back.

We found a great way to coordinate holidays with the kids. One year, they all come home for Thanksgiving, then all go to their in-laws for Christmas. The next year, they go to the in-laws for Thanksgiving, then come home in December. They are away for Thanksgiving this year. So this time, I get to have my wife all to myself.

I got a coronavirus test a few days before I left and again immediately after getting picked up from the airport. By now, I was getting used to that stick shoved up my nose. Well, not really. Again I was negative and had no symptoms.

We kept our distance for a quick minute, but that didn't last very long. We both knew I'd been protected above the CDC guidelines, but we both knew the risk was not zero. I could be asymptomatic and spreading this disease without knowing, or I could be early in the disease process and the virus hasn't replicated enough to be detected by tests. We took full advantage of our five days together, if you know what I mean…

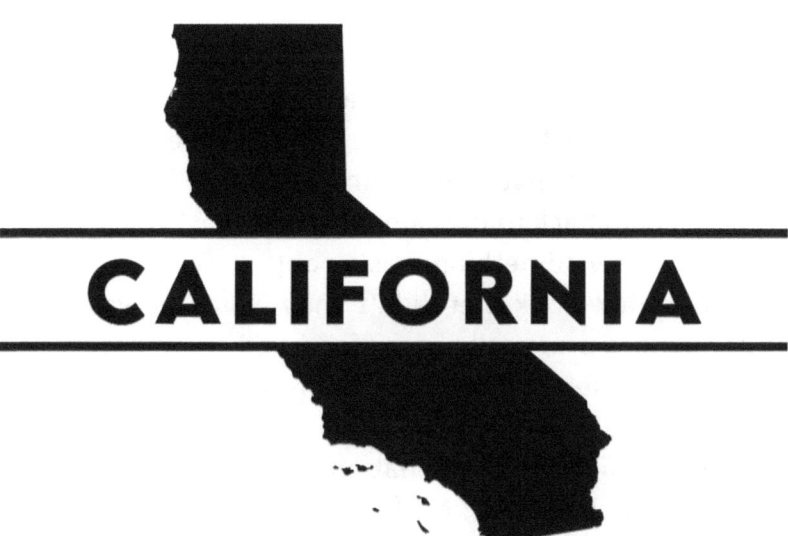

November 29, 2020

I returned to southern California after my short and desperately needed vacation. It was amazing how those few days felt like I had been walking in the desert for a month, baking in the scorching hot sun with no water or food, and then stumbled on an oasis with cool fresh waterfalls, shady palm trees, and fresh succulent fruit hanging low at arm's reach. I only have three weeks left, then I am back home for Christmas.

As I was ironing my scrubs for the week, I started to get a craving for something really delicious. My favorite restaurant close to the hospital has the best blueberry walnut pancakes that were calling my name. I ordered and brought them back to my camper to eat. I ate one bite and instantly knew something was wrong. It seemed like the café got a new cook that didn't know what he was doing. I put my nose practically in my food and could not smell a thing. Then, I felt a stone lurch in my stomach, and I knew it was not the cook. I had a delicious smelling candle in my room and could not smell that either. I did not feel sick at all. No other symptoms. No fever or chills, no body aches, or pain. No nausea or diarrhea. This could not be real! Oh my God! I was infected with coronavirus! I'd been so careful, how could this have happened? I could not believe this.

As I drove to the hospital, I called my wife all freaked out. "Baby! I can't smell anything! I can't taste anything! I got coronavirus and I was just home! How could this happen? How could I be sick?!"

Sandra did not answer because I couldn't stop talking anyway.

"I had my candle burning in the camper and I couldn't smell it! I stuck my nose in my wonderful blueberry pancakes. I couldn't taste it and couldn't smell it. It was like cardboard! But I don't feel sick. I don't have fever or a sore throat or anything!"

"Well, you need to go get tested, but you know what you have. You've got it," she said.

"I'm already driving there. I've been talking so much. How are you doing?"

"I'm sorry to tell you, baby. I'm sick too."

"What!?!" I yelled.

"I have a fever of 103, headache, and body aches. I'm exhausted and in bed."

I couldn't answer. I couldn't breathe! I felt like I started hyperventilating and was dizzy and about to pass out. I put my wife in danger. My best friend! I risked her life by being selfish and going home. For what?! A few days of relaxation? At what price? It definitely was not worth her life!

"One good thing is I'm not short of breath and I'm not coughing, so I'll be alright," Sandra said.

I still couldn't answer her. I visualized myself in a hospital bed in the ICU on a ventilator like all those hundreds of patients I have seen this year. And then I saw my wife twelve hundred miles away in another hospital in a worse predicament than me. Of all places, I never thought I would get it while working at this small rural hospital. It blew my mind. Lots of people think they are fine and end up dying in their bed. Her fever was so high. If she died, I didn't know how I would go on.

I arrived at the hospital and a greater feeling of nervousness overcame me when I was told to drive around back to the ambulance bay to get a confirmation test.

Thoughts of death went through my head; all my patients who died this the year and how their families suffered along with them. I protected myself so well. Yet in the back of my mind, I knew I was immersed for endless hours in disease infected facilities. Eventually it could happen to me. Now it did, and I brought it home to Sandra in her delicate health!

I waited for three of the longest hours of my life sitting in my car outside the ER. I knew the obvious when the ED nurse walked up to my vehicle shaking his head. He said with a little chuckle, "Brother, you are positively positive, sorry man."

I drove away with tears in my eyes and called my wife again. My head was spinning so fast it was hard to drive. What had I done?!? How could I have this? My baby was sick, really sick and all I had was an insane, uncanny complete loss of smell and taste. So far, neither one of us had respiratory symptoms and we didn't need to be in a hospital—yet.

I made it back to my camper and once again, I was quarantined. To be totally honest, I broke down and cried for a long time with swirling thoughts of my sweetheart, the love of my life, actually she is my life, possibly ending up in the ICU on a vent. With her weak immune system, she would be one of those that would start off on a nasal canula, then to BiPAP, then to the ventilator, and you know how that could easily turn out. I cannot lose her.

I don't know how long I was messed up about all this, but finally after a while, I felt I could have a conversation. I called the wonderful couple who rented me the camper and they were floored. They reassured me they would help with anything I needed. I then texted our kids and they promised to help make sure Sandra would manage through this alright. Even though Sandra is a doctor and knows what to do, I also know with her stubborn streak, she would unlikely go to the hospital. She thinks she can manage every situation on her own. I love her independence, but not in situations like this.

I talked with Logan. He and his wife made sure she was hydrating and watched her oxygen level and fever. Logan was surprised when I told him the house of a doctor and a nurse didn't have any meds for fever nor a thermometer. How was she supposed to monitor and take care of herself? Logan managed everything and also put a full liter of water at her bedside. Elise's shift at the fire station just ended and she stopped by to make sure she thought Sandra was well enough to be able to stay at home.

That night I was torn up. I certainly couldn't sleep. Worrying about my wife dying and me going to the ER sent me in a panic with shortness of breath. I called Sandra and I know I woke her up.

"Sandra, were you sleeping?" I asked.

"Yes, but I'm okay," Sandra answered.

"It's probably just a panic attack, but I can't breathe. Should I go to the ER?" I asked.

"Are you coughing?" she asked.

"No," I answered.

"You know all the mucous the coronavirus makes. If you were short of breath because of the virus, you would be coughing. You are panicking. Calm your breathing, baby. Take some deep breaths," she soothed.

"You're making sense. You're right." I started to feel better already.

"Listen hon, I can't talk anymore. I'm exhausted. I got to get off the phone. I gotta go," and she hung up.

She has never hung up on me before and never has she told me she was too sick to talk, even through all that she suffered with her cancer! I jumped up from my chair, paced up and down the camper, crying and screaming, "How could this be happening?! Not her! NO!"

I called Logan again sobbing uncontrollably. It was so hard to get the words out. I asked him to go right then and go check on his mom. I had to go home right now, but how? I couldn't get on a plane, and driving would take way too long. This was so awful. I needed to be with my wife and now!

Logan stayed calm and assured me he would go check on Sandra right away. He kept talking with me as he drove over and saw she was sleeping peacefully. Her oxygen was good, and her temperature was a little lower.

I finally could breathe again. I asked him to not tell anyone I was acting like a baby worrying about my woman. He said he promised. But now, I feel it is a good opportunity to embrace that it's normal for men to cry sometimes. I am a sensitive guy in a tough man's body. If anyone wants to try to make fun or shame me, they are welcome to come talk to my multiple martial arts black belts.

November 30, 2020

I was still in agony over getting the virus and infecting my wife. I was so upset I could not speak with anyone, but her. And she was feeling so bad, she still didn't want to talk, which made me feel worse. As per protocol, I can't do anything and can't go anywhere. I didn't want to anyway; I just stewed over this all day long. The minutes seemed like hours and the hours like days. I texted the kids many times to make sure they were checking on their mom. Of course, they were taking great care of Sandra. I still couldn't think of anything else.

Romy, the lady who owns the camper I was renting, was nice to leave food on the steps for me. She also made me this tonic concoction of turmeric with some other herbs. It made me queasy to look at it, but it was easy to drink since I could not taste anything. She made it with TLC and I needed all I could get right now.

	COVID CASES		COVID DEATHS	
JAN	Global 12,308	US 1	Global 265	US 0
FEB	Global 86,471	US 60	Global 2,978	US 0
MAR	Global 889,005	US 149,378	Global 45,236	US 5,210
APR	Global 3,482,232	US 1,086,625	Global 238,993	US 62,955
MAY	Global 6,515,313	US 1,856,560	Global 382,743	US 108,439
JUN	Global 10,575,194	US 2,762,809	Global 526,357	US 129,710
JUL	Global 17,627,792	US 4,708,945	Global 694,078	US 157,386
AUG	Global 26,012,690	US 6,234,482	Global 866,636	US 187,596
SEP	Global 34,891,132	US 7,532,411	Global 1,020,526	US 212,082
OCT	Global 47,161,108	US 9,395,274	Global 1,202,691	US 235,492
NOV	Global 63,485,398	US 13,998,001	Global 1,474,878	US 273,023

December 1, 2020

I didn't want to bother Sandra, but I needed to know how she was every single hour. If I could, I would have had a video monitor on to watch her every minute. I was so worried for her. And for me if I lost her.

So far, I hadn't gotten any worse, so I might make it through without further complications. Sandra assured me she was feeling better, but I was not convinced. People have been seriously sick at home for days and then just don't wake up. Or when they finally decide to go to the hospital, it's too late. This could happen to her. This anguish reminded me of the torture I went through with my dad.

My pop was known as Reverend Street. He was a prominent member of the little community where we lived. Whenever I think about that man, I feel my heart get bigger with tremendous love for him. He will always be my hero. If we drove by a car that was broken down alongside the road, my father always stopped to help. He helped everyone! I don't know how he had the time for all that. To this day, I can never figure out how hard he worked at that shipyard and still made time to put his sermons together for church every Sunday. I also never discovered how he found any time left to spend with each and every one of my seven sisters and three brothers, yet he did.

This great man died on December 4, 2012 with ALS (Lou Gehrig's disease). While there are those who last several years, my pop went fast. Some say that was a blessing. But it was a double-edged sword, because he left us too soon. In good health, he was 5 foot 9 inches and weighed 180 pounds. After his diagnosis, he dropped to eighty pounds in one year. There hasn't been a worse moment for my family. I still cry when I talk about him.

I tried to go home as often as I could, and it made me smile to see how he was comforted with my visits. I guess he felt safe with me being a nurse because I could handle a medical situation if it came up. One of the last times I was with my pop was when we took him to the ER for aspiration. When he could not swallow his own spit, he panicked something awful and his saliva would go down the wrong tube. The ED doc hydrated him and gave him some oxygen. He was discharged to go home once he started feeling better.

As we walked out, he slowly turned to face a crowded waiting room of about fifteen to twenty people. He could barely stand up, but he wanted to walk anyway. I held him on his right side under his armpit and my momma held him around his waist on the left. He looked at the strangers and said, "God loves each and every one of you, and so do I. May God bless you all. I will pray for you." My momma and I broke down in tears as we walked out. He taught me to love thy neighbor as a brother and to show love to everyone no matter what, even if they steal my money or say horrible things about me. I'm proud to be that preacher's son.

I know Sandra would have loved my pop. It's sad she never got to meet him. There are things about her that remind me of him. She and her sister also grew up in a religious home with their father who is a preacher man. It's true what they say about preacher's children. No, they are not all hell raisers (although some definitely are). They have strong kind hearts.

December 2, 2020

Another restless night. I didn't expect any different. My love was sick with the virus and so far away. I couldn't drive to her. She was still assuring me she was not getting any worse. Sandra tried to make me laugh to distract me, so she told me about some things going on in the world. She lived in New

Orleans for more than twenty years when she was younger, so she keeps up with the news from there.

Most of us adults have heard of swingers. If you are swinging, that is your free choice. However, when a leader of a city gives permission to throw a big swinging conference during a global COVID outbreak, I wonder how they came to that decision. The Mayor of New Orleans allowed "Naughty in N'Awlins" to take place. Not for a few hours, or a day, but for four consecutive days starting Nov 11. While normally two thousand people attend, this year there was a scant two hundred fifty.

Sure, there was required social distancing with couples having to stay at their own tables. They waved their hankies in the air standing in place pretending to "second-line" dance. And I would almost bet you this party was not just cocktails and caviar. Even if they were separated at the group events, what happened after those 250 people left? Did they all go home or to their hotels without swapping or swinging? The virus is spread through respiratory droplets and contact, as everyone on the planet must know by now. I guarantee you there was a lot of contact and respiratory droplets exchanged during this conference. COVID...the new STD?

On February 25 over 500,000 folks attended Mardi Gras in New Orleans. Understandably, the Mayor went by what the Trump administration was saying that there was nothing to be worried about—the virus was contained in the US. So, she allowed the event to happen. Two weeks later, the first COVID case emerged in Louisiana. Then a few days after that it was like a coronavirus bomb exploding.

Sandra told me about a cell phone location map showing lights spreading across the US representing people who attended the festivities this year and where they traveled afterwards. Then more dots lit up showing the positive COVID cases that resulted. It was terrifying to see how those lights mushroomed across America so quickly like an electronic board game.

December 4, 2020

I called Sandra. I could hear in her voice she was starting to feel better. My heart began to smile again. I couldn't imagine being without my baby, my rock, my hero, my everything. I thought I was whole when I met her. But then that's when I realized I was half a person without her. She is the air that makes me breathe easier. Now I can relax a little bit, knowing that her fever was down, and her oxygen was mid to upper 90s. We still have a ways to go before she's really out of danger. I hope the aches and fatigue will leave her soon.

I didn't plan on arriving to immediately get quarantined. I was intending on going to the grocery store the day I got those pancakes and Miss Rona put a stop to that. Being the wonderful wife she is, Sandra gave me a good solution for my dilemma for groceries. She suggested I order my food online and drive to the curbside pick-up area. When the delivery guy comes out, I can pop the trunk. There's no need to get anywhere near anyone. She is so smart! I guess I am smart, too. I asked her to marry me.

Today was also the sad anniversary of the death of my pop. Since this camper is in a remote neighborhood on a mountain, it's essentially isolated. I took a long walk alone with nature and didn't see anyone. I usually feel him with me a lot, but I felt him especially strongly today. I thought of all the stories he told me, the lessons I learned from him, the attention he showed each one of us kids. He was respected and loved by the entire community. I knew he would have enjoyed this beauty all around me. I am sure he is with me in spirit.

December 6, 2020

Going outside in the sunshine helped me from going nuts in this quarantine. The long walks brought me back to those days when I was in the best shape of my life in Oman. Since we couldn't leave the base, we had to come up with our own recreations. We were certain our activities would not have the same bad side effects like a poor soldier who came into the base hospital with a serious Gonorrhea infection in his eye from his "diversions".

We came up with a monthly Strong Man Competition. Troops volunteered to compete against each other in this timed event demonstrating superhuman strength. The prize was $300, along with the honor of having the title The Best of the Best on the base.

The Humvee Pull was where the contestant planted himself a hundred feet away and had to pull a Humvee to him using a two-inch rope. Next, we had to flip a big tractor tire from one end of the sand volleyball court to the other. Then, we had to place increasing weight dumbbells from sixty to one hundred twenty pounds on gradually higher steps made from pallets. After finishing all of that, we were completely fatigued, but we were far from done.

In the fireman's obstacle, we sprinted thirty feet to reach a 180-pound dummy. We had to either drag or carry it to safety for another thirty feet. In that safety zone there was a rolled-up fire hose that we had to grab and unroll as we ran back to the starting point. The objective was to open the water valve and control that hose while filling a five-gallon bucket fifty feet away.

The next station was two ten-foot-long railroad ties placed parallel to each other with a space just large enough for a shorter five foot section to slide between. Standing on the two longer ties, we swung a sledgehammer hitting the shorter tie moving it the entire ten-foot length.

The last event was reminiscent of the days when a prisoner had his arms tied to two horses facing in opposite directions. Two Evil Knievel like jump ramps were placed about ten feet apart. A four-wheeler was driven to the top of each ramp. The driver put it in neutral and squeezed the brakes, so the vehicle would not roll back. The contestant stood on the ground in the middle between the two ramps holding straps connected to the front bumper of the two ATVs. When the contestant was in place, the drivers let go of the brakes and the four-wheelers started sliding backwards. We held on as long as we could to keep the ATVs from rolling back down the ramp. Eventually, we had to let go or get our shoulders dislocated.

After all those exhausting events were performed as fast as we possibly could, we had to sprint one mile on a treadmill. This competition with all these ridiculously macho events energized the entire base, contestants, and spectators alike. It is one of my favorite memories of my military days.

I felt like one of those winners today because Sandra was feeling much better. I know she'll make it out fine. Now, I can actually see and think straight. These have been the worst days, thinking I might lose her and so close to the anniversary of my pop's death. I don't think I could live with that. It was mind boggling that I couldn't be with her when she was sick. I'm glad our kids are always so wonderful and helpful.

December 9, 2020

I still had no other symptoms other than not being able to smell or taste. It was such a weird thing. And knowing I couldn't taste food made me think about how my mouth used to water while smelling aromas of delicious dishes.

I grew up with seven sisters who all knew how to cook, and even my brothers could throw down in the kitchen. Everyone thinks their momma is the best cook, well my momma IS the best cook on the planet. I remember the days growing up in Basin, Mississippi when my two youngest sisters and I would race to the end of our dirt road to meet our pop coming home from the shipyard. Our pop had this musky smell all the time, which was not a stinky smell, it was a manly smell. I'm sure it was his natural testosterone that made my pop seem superhuman. He was also a handsome man, so you can only imagine what those church-going women thought when he got up to preach on Sundays. He was also a Scorpio, like me. If you know zodiac signs, then you understand where I'm going.

Anyway, we would race to the end of the road to see who could get to his leftover peanut butter and jelly sandwiches or that can of leftover Vienna sausages. I believe he brought them home just for us because he knew how much we enjoyed it. This was every weekday of my young boyhood. Sometimes he would have a pack of spearmint or double mint gum. I could smell the scent of the gum busting through his musk and we knew he was going to give us all a stick. We were so happy and proud of our daddy.

My momma was our hero, too. She is that strong super woman that made magic happen around our family. She made sure to make her husband proud and happy, like my wife does with me. We grew up in a strong, loving, and happy home. I feel so blessed because not all people grow up in this happiness. As we walked up to our front porch jumping and pawing on pop, we could smell the delicious food breaking through the fresh smell of pine cleaner on newly mopped hard wood floors. That soul food—collard greens, fried chicken, red beans and rice, and sweet corn bread—I can eat this every day. Country folk know what I'm talking about.

Now I can cook. Years ago, I went to a culinary art school on a fifteen-week program just to learn more about the art of cooking. When I first met my wife, she worked at hospitals where she had to stay overnight for seven consecutive days every few weeks. I would bring her lunch and dinner. She loved my cooking, like most folks who have tasted my food. Well, let me tell you something—shortly after my wife and I started dating, she made the mistake she regrets to this very day. She gave me a break in the kitchen and whipped up an amazing Shrimp Creole out of nothing. Oh my God, she cooks like someone's momma—like my momma. Damn, I am one lucky man. I got double the momma's cooking, which makes my cuisine taste like garbage. Some folks work magic in the kitchen. It's their laboratory where formulas and recipes are the blank canvas, and spices and herbs are their tools to create a masterpiece that will take your taste buds where they have never been before. Hell, I discovered taste buds I never knew I had until I ate my wife's food. I don't know if it's because she's Brazilian, or if it's genetics, or just another freaking level of genius in her.

Dec 11, 2020

Romy has left me those funky looking herbal tonics every day. I drank them because she took the time and care to make them for me. I also know as bad as they looked, they had to be healthy. As my sense of taste and smell started to come back, I discovered they were one of the best tasting drinks I've ever had. I have to get her recipe.

The CDC has loosened the guidelines for asymptomatic healthcare workers. I was only banished for ten days instead of two full weeks. I am done with my second quarantine. With the vaccine coming, hopefully, there won't be another one. To celebrate, I went to visit Louis at Kämənz Kafé, and devoured a fantastic turkey ciabatta sandwich along with my favorite honey lavender latte. This was a real experience! I smelled every nuance and smothered my taste buds in all that goodness.

December 12, 2020

When I got to work, people were happy to see me. There were a lot of hospital staff who tested positive and were out sick. In addition to this, there were a great many patients and we were well over capacity. Since COVID was hitting home, people were scared.

Co-workers were curious about my symptoms. They were amazed at how mild of a case I had. Thankfully my loss of smell and taste was slowly returning back to normal. Since I hardly had any symptoms, in the back of my mind I started to doubt if I had the natural immunity scientists talked about. Am I really protected? I still plan to wear my N95 and PAPR in the hospital as usual. In the community, I'll continue to wear an N95 wherever I go.

The small hospital in this rural town was overflowing with COVID patients now. The surge had begun. Many areas were converted specifically into COVID wards and those rooms were filled to double capacity. ICU spilled over into Med Surg with vented patients in rooms not designed for the critically ill. With many staff out sick, we were all working beyond our normal expectations. To help with the patient load, the hospital hired six more travel nurses for the ICU. I was able to float to areas of the hospital that needed my help. The ER was the area most affected with staff getting exposed. Naturally this was where we had the majority of vacancies on the schedule, so that's where I worked.

We heard on the scanner there was an accident on Highway 58. One passenger walked away essentially unharmed, but the driver came in by ambulance. He was a 38-year-old with five fractured ribs and evidence of a significant brain injury from alcohol with a BAL almost 500. It was amazing he was still breathing with that much alcohol on board. He was also COVID-positive and interestingly enough, he had a blood clot in his leg. We see clots with COVID, but they are unusual in alcoholics because they tend to bleed due to having low platelets from liver disease.

The patient was increasingly lethargic and continued to deteriorate. The alcohol had poisoned his brain and we knew he needed more than we could offer in this remote hospital. We do not have Neuro specialists and with COVID surging in Southern California, it was hard to get him to the appropriate place. After a few days, we finally were able to transfer him to a larger facility to get the specialized care he needed. We found out he caught COVID from a gathering with his family and friends. Unfortunately, we heard he died two days later from his alcohol abuse and the usual complications of his COVID infection.

December 18, 2020

I got the first dose of my vaccine today. It was documented with photos and video to be aired during the holidays across the nation on an interview with CBS. This media attention was to help people feel good about getting the shot. All the medical staff at this local hospital would gladly offer their arm to take it.

Now, the shot itself could have side effects, but I promise it won't turn you into a lizard or your skin won't grow scales like the Brazilian president suggested. After my injection, my arm was sore, and I felt feverish and achy. I took acetaminophen (Tylenol) for my symptoms and they went away.

It is important to debunk the great amount of misinformation and help all people understand what is really going on in the coronavirus world. I appeal especially to people of color to gain confidence to get vaccinated. There are many aspects that have led to this point of distrust and suspicion. Americans on a broad scale have had a gradual deterioration of their trust in our government. We heard the President say in March this virus was contained and for the "vast majority of Americans, the risk is very, very low." Those of us working in hospitals were seeing a very different story.

There had been ridiculous claims on social media saying the vaccine would kill or sterilize certain ethnic groups, or it would alter one's DNA, and even that it was a way the government could insert a microchip tracker into our bloodstream to deposit "nano transducers" in our brains. Come on, people! I get that you may not trust your government, but these claims are too farfetched and nonsensical.

Look at the science. My son is getting his PhD in Molecular Biology. He understands how this vaccine was developed and even though it was done quickly, it was done right. When our bodies get attacked by a virus for the first time, our cells have to learn how to fight it. They can identify a protein or "antigen" on the outside of the virus and start making "antibodies" as soldiers to go kill it. But this natural process takes time. And in that time, the virus continues to multiply, and people get sick.

Vaccines teach your immune system how to fight a specific virus. By teaching the system what the virus looks like beforehand, it can be ready to act quickly. Then if you come into contact with that awful virus, your body knows how to attack it immediately. The vaccine does not cover you 100%. You may still get sick, like some may get a mild case of the flu during flu season, even if they got a flu shot. But they won't get nearly as sick as they would have without it. This vaccine can literally save your life!

December 20, 2020

There are a lot of people in their 70s and 80s who think they can do as much as they did in their 50s. This is because age related deterioration gradually happens over time. It's like you look in the mirror every day and don't see what you would in a photo album of how your picture has changed over the years.

A 76-year-old man was admitted to the hospital yesterday for generalized weakness and anemia. He was helped to a chair so he could eat breakfast and was told not to get up without calling the nurse to ask for assistance. This man did not listen.

After he finished his meal, he pushed his tray table to the side, and proceeded to try to get back into the bed himself. His door was open, so I saw him getting up with his mask dangling from one ear. As I ran to the room, he staggered and caught himself leaning over his freshly made bed with his knees pressed up against the mattress. As I approached him, he came to a standing position and something plopped out of his mouth. I looked on the draw sheet and saw a molar (with root still intact) lying in the middle of the bed. It fell out of his mouth and landed onto the military tucked, quarter bouncing sheets.

"Sir, you just lost a tooth!" I exclaimed.

He responded, "I've been losing all my teeth over the past few years. Now I can't chew food much anymore. I can't eat meat and I've lost a lot of weight."

I said, "Maybe that's one of the reasons you are weak and anemic. We can get the dietician to help you with a good meal plan with soft but healthy foods. In the meantime, what should we do with this tooth? Would you like me to put it under your pillow? I hear the Tooth Fairy still makes house calls here at this hospital."

He laughed as I slowly rotated him to a sitting position onto his bed. We took his tooth and put it in a specimen cup. I contacted the doctor right away. The patient now had a huge hole in his mouth. His history of losing many teeth over several years told me he had gingivitis with an overabundance of bacteria that could lead to a heart valve infection, sepsis, and eventually his demise. Dental hygiene is a very important aspect of overall health. I reminded him to floss at least once a day (it could prevent heart disease) and brush his teeth after every meal. This "Tooth Fairy" ended up bringing the patient intravenous antibiotics for treatment of his tooth decay.

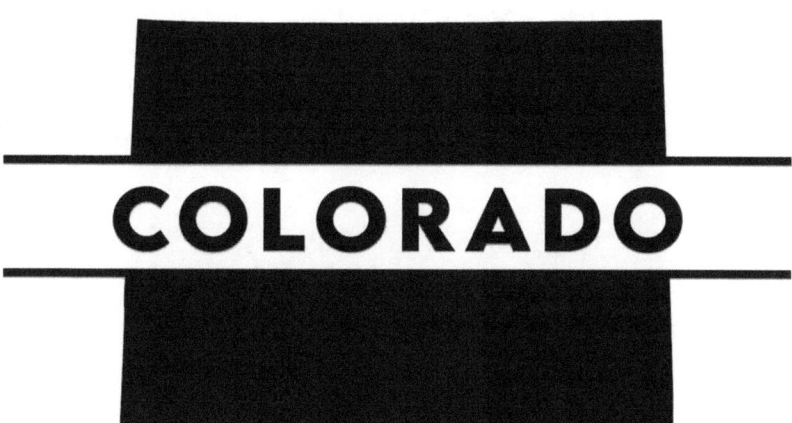

December 22, 2020

My last shift was yesterday, and I am now home for the holidays. It was a long sixteen-hour drive starting early in the morning, but I made it in one day to surprise my wife. As I drove up, I saw that she actually surprised me with holiday lights all around outside. There was the warm glow of icicle lights dripping from the gutters and a beautiful red and green holly garland framing our front door with an elegant wreath in the middle. It was amazing how immediately it worked wonders in warming my heart and removed the sluggish road grime from my brain. She met me at the door with a big smile and a twinkle in her eye…hmmm, I wondered what she had planned for me tonight? We both recently had COVID. Having "natural immunity" for a short while meant no quarantining for me!

December 23, 2020

I had a short "honey-do" list since the kids were coming home for the weekend. There was some cleaning to do around the house, a few last-minute shopping items to buy, and guest rooms to freshen up. Despite the holiday cheer, we both were concerned about new strains of COVID that started popping up around the globe. It was unclear just how much our natural protection would keep us safe with these COVID variants.

Sandra and I have "soldiers" that have seen the virus once and our immune system stands ready and waiting for the next war. The tricky part is that all viruses mutate, changing to adapt to their environment. We do not know yet if our immunity or the vaccine can adequately fight these new strains. It seems like we've been in this pandemic forever, but this virus only began twelve months ago. It is absolutely amazing what scientists have been able to accomplish in such a short time.

Jacob explained it to me very well. Vaccines work the same way that our bodies work. Usual vaccines, like the flu shot, are made from a live but weakened virus (nasal spray), or a small part of a dead virus or the lab makes something that "looks" like the virus. This is injected into the body and our immune system starts to make antibodies. The COVID vaccines are a little different and most scientists feel they are actually safer. The technique of using mRNA is one that scientists have been studying and working with for many years. That is why they were able to double-down their efforts and have a vaccine using this new technique in such a short time.

mRNA sounds a lot like DNA and that has stirred up many misconceptions. Our bodies use mRNA as simple coders or messengers, giving our cells basic instructions on what to do. These new vaccines carry an mRNA with one simple message—for our own human cells to make a version of that virus protein to educate the immune system on coronavirus. This human-made protein is not the virus. You cannot get COVID from it.

Anytime the immune system reacts, you may have fever, body aches, or fatigue. This means you are making your "platoons of soldiers" to prepare for a real exposure. The mRNA only carries that one specific order, to make that protein. No other codes exist to change our DNA. No other codes can turn us into lizard mutants or make us radioactive.

Those theories are ridiculous and not even good to use in a B-rated sci-fi movie.

We saw on the news that a doctor in Florida died from a brain bleed a few days after taking the vaccine. His body stopped making platelets and an artery started leaking. This was extremely sad and unfortunate. The MMR vaccine we freely give our children has this same and very rare risk as well. Nine million people to date have had the COVID vaccine with only twenty-nine severe allergic reactions, and that was the only reported death. So, my thought is this—are your chances of dying higher with the vaccine, or higher if you actually get COVID?

We all think about our mortality from time to time. It would be great if we could pick the manner in which we go to the great beyond. Most would choose to go peacefully in the night. I would rather die by hanging, or burning at the stake, or drowning, than to die in the way hundreds of people I have seen die from this horrible disease. Any death is faster with much less collective suffering. The sad part of all is many COVID deaths are preventable. #wearamask #sanitizeyourhands #socialdistance #getvaccinated

December 26, 2020

Elise was on shift on Christmas Day, so we celebrated this weekend. Logan and Kaitlyn live ten minutes away and came early for breakfast. We made lattes and pecan-craisin waffles with made-to-order omelets while we waited for Jacob and Hallie to drive in from Wyoming. They all wore cloth masks while my wife and I wore N95s. We stayed as distant as possible, at least six to ten feet away from one another. We were determined not to have a repeat of the Thanksgiving horror. We certainly did not want a second round with a different strain.

While lunch was cooking in the oven, wonderful smells filled the air, and sounds of holiday instrumental music surrounded us. We took that time to get caught up on the recent events in our kids' lives. After opening presents, we finished cooking together and ate again.

Since the weather was so nice, we took a walk in the neighborhood to help us make room for dessert. Isn't it so funny how on the holidays we eat and eat, then cook to eat some more? We played board games, laughed, and joked, then called Sandra's sister in Hawai'i. Every year we think about her hanging ornaments on a palm tree. I guess her version of a white Christmas is with sand on a beach. Not quite the same to me.

The hospital in southern California texted several times since I've been home, asking if I would consider going back. It's not even New Year's yet. I got emails almost daily with hundreds of nursing spots open across the country. Hospitals were begging for help. We know the time frame for a surge is about two weeks after a holiday. With Christmas and New Year one week apart, mid-January it will hit and hit hard. That is when I will plan to go somewhere.

For now, I didn't want to spend my time thinking about leaving already. I wanted to concentrate on my wife and kids, enjoying homemade lattes in the morning, doing projects around the house, snuggling in front of the fireplace in the evenings while watching a good movie and eating popcorn, and best of all, restfully sleeping in my comfy bed next to my amazing Sandra. I feel so lucky to be where I am today and who is with me. What a life!

December 31, 2020

There are hundreds of assignments in so many states, it's hard to figure out where to go next. I was considering New York or New Jersey again. There are also many jobs across the South and Midwest. My previous supervisor in southern California was still texting for me to return. I asked my wife her opinion. Of course, she wanted me to go back to the small hospital in rural California. She said, "They need your help, baby. You have so much experience with hospitals overrun with COVID and those nurses will be overwhelmed with the post-holiday surge by mid-January. You also know all those nice people already, along with the workflow of the hospital. It will be easy and comfortable for you to return to a familiar place." As always, she is right.

New Year's Eve was upon us. The kids were planning small get-togethers with their friends. As for my wife and me, we planned to celebrate in pandemic fashion and watch a feel-good film until the ball dropped online. First, we had the cancer year of 2019, then the COVID crisis in 2020. This new year of 2021 is bound to be better!

	COVID CASES		COVID DEATHS	
JAN	Global 12,308	US 1	Global 265	US 0
FEB	Global 86,471	US 60	Global 2,978	US 0
MAR	Global 889,005	US 149,378	Global 45,236	US 5,210
APR	Global 3,482,232	US 1,086,625	Global 238,993	US 62,955
MAY	Global 6,515,313	US 1,856,560	Global 382,743	US 108,439
JUN	Global 10,575,194	US 2,762,809	Global 526,357	US 129,710
JUL	Global 17,627,792	US 4,708,945	Global 694,078	US 157,386
AUG	Global 26,012,690	US 6,234,482	Global 866,636	US 187,596
SEP	Global 34,891,132	US 7,532,411	Global 1,020,526	US 212,082
OCT	Global 47,161,108	US 9,395,274	Global 1,202,691	US 235,492
NOV	Global 63,485,398	US 13,998,001	Global 1,474,878	US 273,023
DEC	Global 83,943,230	US 20,502,143	Global 1,797,727	US 354,391

January 1, 2021

New Year's Day was quiet at the house. Sandra and I enjoyed each other's company talking about the past two years of upheaval with her cancer and the pandemic. We ruminated on what the future could hold for us and our family. Instead of the traditional southern New Year's good luck meal of cabbage and black-eyed peas, we spent a lot of time in the kitchen making a Cajun gumbo celebration. Sandra made the roux, since she says I never cook mine long enough. It is usual to use Gumbo File in every self-respecting Southerner's gumbo. Unfortunately, Sandra reacts with a horrible stuffed up nose and itchy throat, so that is out. Since we are in Colorado, fresh okra is not an easy find this time of year, so frozen would have to work.

It would be really great if we could take those vacations this year. At least we know our enemy and how to combat it. I wish others would cooperate, so we can get closer to a normal life before we forget what that is like. It will be much easier to travel once we are all vaccinated.

January 6, 2021

There were tears in my eyes today because at the worst time in our country's history as we face this deadly global pandemic, we had leadership constantly downplaying the dangers of this virus, discounting the recommendations of top scientists, and now supporting White supremacists inciting a coup against democracy. It hurt me deep in my soul when I saw the videos of the riots that happened at the Capitol, with White supremacists in the midst. It reminded me of those old news clips from the 50s and 60s when folks were beaten by cops and racist White people in the South during the civil rights movement.

Regardless of whether you are on the side of the red or blue, we all enjoy the freedoms that come with democracy. Remember the Preamble to the Constitution, "We the people of the United States, in order to form a more perfect union, establish justice, ensure domestic tranquility, provide for the common defense, promote the general welfare, and secure the blessings of liberty to ourselves and our posterity, do ordain and establish this Constitution for the United States of America."

The Preamble broken down in my simple words is for us to come together as people in unity. Let us respect and protect each other, especially during this time of a world tragedy and not create additional national crises. We can live or go to school where we want. We can choose any profession or completely change directions at any time. We can buy a car, any car. We can sell our house for the going rate in the market, not at a predetermined price set by the government. We can even decide how many children we want to have or to have none at all.

The events that occurred today were a travesty to our country. After a fair election, proven over sixty times in court, some citizens of this great country felt it was their right to try and overturn our newly elected president. They violently tried taking control of the highest seat of government just because their candidate did not win. It sent chills all over my body at how close we came to losing our freedom. We had divisive leadership encouraging a coup in response to a fair democratic election loss. Americans died as a result and will continue dying if something is not done.

Everyone I know on both sides of the political fence is shocked and embarrassed a coup was attempted in this country by our own people. We cannot let this type of immoral anarchy to succeed—ever. We vote as American citizens and must live with the results, whatever they are. We must humbly win and graciously lose.

Democracy is defined as a "system of government by the people, especially a rule of the majority. It is a government in which the supreme power is vested in the people and exercised by them directly or indirectly through a system of representation usually involving periodically held free elections." This is how we base our current freedom.

The highest court in our land, the Supreme Court, reviewed and decided twice the election was fair. There was no basis to overturn the result. A recount maintained the truly elected leader. Our nation needs to heal its wounds and work together, regardless of personal bias.

Let us unite as American people no matter the color of our skin or our chosen political affiliation. Let us appreciate our different heritages, realizing that is what makes our country so special. The United States of America once was the greatest country in the world. We have fallen far from that by internal division over politics, race, ethnic background, sexual orientation, and gender. United we can build to be stronger than we once were.

January 7, 2021

I needed my booster vaccine and had to find a place here to get the second one on time. I use the VA for my healthcare as a disabled war vet. I tried there first, since they have vaccines. I was told for documentation purposes, that I really should get the booster at the same location as my first. But I would be out of the twenty-one-day window when I return to Tehachapi and could not wait that long. After a few days of internal discussions at the VA, they made an exception, and gave me the second shot. From everything I heard, I was expecting to have more symptoms than before. Because my body was partially primed, there was a greater chance for a reaction. I was surprised to have not one ache, pain, or fever.

Jan 12, 2021

The news was still non-stop with all the political mess. I heard a reporter say she's overused the word unprecedented in the last year. And it's the sad truth. That word is applicable not just with a global pandemic, but with our political division, our racial conflicts being brought to center stage, and also for the recent climate extremes around the globe. I wonder when all this will settle.

January 16, 2021

I got up well before the break of day, took a shower, got dressed, and sat with my wife and our coffees for one last time before I hit the road. It would take about sixteen hours to get to California. Most of the trip, I had reception and talked for hours with my love to keep me awake. It is so funny how since I was young, I always hated to talk on the phone. My dad was the same way. It is like drinking cod liver oil to me. Yet I can talk to my wife all day long, never get tired of it, and never run out of things to say.

While I was driving, Sandra called and told me her father, Dylton, tested positive for COVID-19. His wife, Lane, was surprisingly negative. She has severe dementia, so her daughters drove her two and a half hours away from Houston to the vacant house of her long time ago ex-husband, who died a few months prior. Lane is a sweet mild-mannered woman and was confused about being in a strange house alone and unable to have visitors. She didn't understand why her husband couldn't be with her or come to pick her up to return home. Sandra talked with her father and felt his symptoms were mild enough and he was competent enough to stay isolated without assistance, for now. Being older, Dylton is at a great risk and his condition could worsen very quickly.

He told us the story about how he contracted the virus. He had a friend who was isolating in a hotel with COVID. Dylton brought food to him a few times and placed the package near the door. He always wore a mask and stepped back six to eight feet. The sick man opened the door to say hello and joined in a prayer to God for healing. On two occasions, the man did not wear a mask and was coughing. A threshold of an open doorway is not a magical barrier where if you don't cross your toe over it you can't infect another. It is unbelievable the man didn't put on a mask before opening the door. Dylton could have immediately left or asked him to cover his face. They could have talked through the closed door or outside a window. This was 100% preventable. I hope they all survive this.

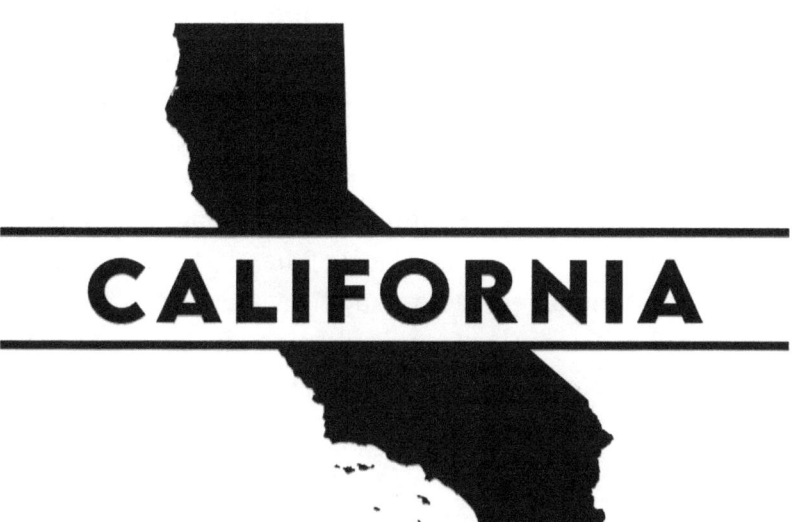

January 17, 2021

I finally arrived in California and unloaded my bags. I plan to go tomorrow to shop for weekly groceries, then wash and gas up my car. But tonight, I was tired and got Chinese fast food. This town is so small that it was not unusual to run into someone I know. I saw a nurse who works at the hospital and she told me everyone was excited I was back. There were so many sick patients they had ICU overflowing on the regular unit. The issue with that is those rooms are smaller and not big enough for all the equipment needed to adequately care for the critically ill. Also, there are none of the usual ICU sophisticated machines and not enough heart monitors to put on the patients. She told me to expect to work twelve to sixteen hours each day and at least six days every week, maybe seven. I worked like that in Miami at a much larger hospital and managed to do okay. There wouldn't be much time to talk to Sandra, but we would manage. I got my supper ready, then prepared for our date night—1200 miles apart.

January 18, 2021

In this second assignment the hospital looked entirely different than it did in December. As soon as I drove up, the full parking lot surprised me. I have never seen so many people at this little hospital in this little town. At least I didn't see a big triage tent with a line of people wrapped around the building like in New Jersey.

I am here in the trenches and see the dilemma faced by hospital administration. It's important to keep known COVID patients separated from non-COVID patients. That part is easy, if you know who is positive and if there is no limit to the size of the building. But what if a patient comes in with symptoms and their COVID status is not yet known? We see them in the ED and get the test. Where do they wait while the test is being run? In the room with COVID patients? What if their test comes back negative? Do we put them in the non-COVID waiting room? What if the test returns positive and they just exposed everyone? There is just not enough space to keep everyone in private rooms, separated by walls, or a closed door. Other hospitals around the country ask patients to wait in their vehicles until the test results are finalized. That is okay if they are not that sick. The real issue is they cannot wait with portable oxygen or be attached to an IV pole with fluids hanging in their cars. Since we are out of space, that is the best we can do.

This is a world-wide pandemic and we are the hardest hit with rising numbers far exceeding any other country. As residents of the "first-world" United States, we are all used to the best of the best. But now we are in a war zone and our "first-world" perspective needs to adjust to the harsh reality in which we are now living.

January 19, 2021

I heard some healthcare workers here were not getting the vaccine. Instead, they elected to wait to see how others would do. I also heard there were hospitals in some southern states that still had thousands of doses left in their refrigerators because 70-80% of their staff were refusing to get vaccinated. What the heck, people?! It makes no sense to me why we aren't all chasing the vaccine.

First, people complain that the government stay-at-home orders are shutting down our economy. This is to protect the community from this deadly virus and to reduce the potential spread by decreasing the mingling of people during times of high viral propagation. Then there are complaints about having to wear masks in public and practice social distancing under the pretense that the government is invading individual civil rights. Are seatbelt laws and traffic speed limits similar invasions of personal rights as well? Now people are deciding to boycott the vaccine due to fear that it is more dangerous to get the vaccine than to die from COVID.

The hesitancy to get the vaccine is much more prevalent in minorities than in Whites. They see the government as mostly White men in charge, making the rules to their own advantage. We can see evidence of this in the economic disparity between the races that range from unemployment to professional salaries. People of color are hired less often and make less money than their White counterparts. The data out there is unbiased and clear. This distrust of the government of this great country in which we live fuels the fire that consumes our sense of reason about this pandemic. Many have lost their faith in their government and in the lifesaving fluid in the vaccine syringe.

The suspicion of the vaccine is not only isolated to minority groups. Whites and Blacks alike are worried that the vaccine was developed too fast, making it unsafe. Both groups are also concerned that the virus is changing rapidly, and the vaccine may not work against new strains. These are reasonable fears. But people still get on a plane even though they may have a fear of flying. They trust the pilot is educated and trained to defy gravity and fly a heavy metal machine to a destination and get everyone safely on the ground. We must now put our faith in the professionals who are educated and trained to develop these vaccines. I hope everyone looks at this with a scientific mind, instead of with political emotion, so we can move on from this crisis as a society.

Vaccines are essential to get control of this pandemic, because if everyone's immune system is prepared to fight this virus, it won't be able to grow and spread through a population easily like we are seeing with this historic disaster. Think of it like when the European explorers went to the New World. They exposed native people to all sorts of illnesses to which they had no immunity and they died in hordes. This is kind of what is happening to us now.

As a global society, we have lost so much to COVID-19. To win this war, we need to band together against this common enemy and do everything in our power to overcome. We all need to wear our masks in public, out of courtesy and respect for one another. We need to stay socially distant, as much as the situations will allow. We need to sanitize our hands before touching our faces as well as before touching anyone else. We need to get the vaccine to slow and eventually stop the spread of this devastating infection.

When I finished my shift, I called Sandra on my way back to my apartment. She told me that Lane was now sick. She had been staying by herself with one of her daughters coming in to heat up food to make sure she ate. She started coughing more than her usual cough, so her daughter took her to get tested. It was no surprise to learn she was now positive. Even though we are not happy she has COVID, it seems to be simpler because her husband could come stay with her. She would be much calmer if she and Dylton could be in the same house, but also be closer to Lane's daughters, so they could bring them food. But Dylton was feeling too sick today to take the long trip to be near his wife.

January 20, 2021

One of the saddest things is to have a loved one in the hospital and none of the family can visit. This is especially difficult when the person is critically ill and expected to die. Our ICU is on the ground floor of this hospital. Families became creative in the ways they tried to communicate. They know the room number of their family and with a little ingenuity they figure out which window is the right one. We saw written messages on some windows of love and support. So much sadness. So much loss.

Coronavirus has changed almost every aspect of our world. The grieving process is no exception. Families cannot say good-bye and cannot hold their dear one's hand. Some have not seen their families in months. This hospital has thought outside the box with this situation. When a baby is born, there is a tradition of obtaining their footprint for identification, but also as a nostalgic keepsake of that momentous day.

This hospital is now taking the handprint of the patient using colorful water-based paint. They give that to the family along with a heartfelt message signed by the healthcare team as a last remembrance of the departed. In this horrifically challenging time, the best aspects of humanity still seem to overcome the worst.

One 70-year-old patient died today—one of the lucky ones to have family at his bedside. The man was admitted for shortness of breath due to COVID. We all know the family because his daughter is one of our receptionists. This town is small, and everybody knows everyone else. There is a strict hospital policy no family is allowed in to visit, but this is also her place of work. She did her job diligently and at lunch or breaks, she checked on her dad every day. He lasted about two weeks, which is the trend we are seeing here. It was comforting to his daughter that she could be with him at the end, holding his hand and saying her last goodbyes. She knows how rare it is these days.

Today was the inauguration of President Biden. In a show of solidarity, three former presidents addressed the people of the United States in a call for unity. Two were Democrats and one Republican. Former Presidents Bush, Clinton, and Obama stressed the importance to come together as a nation regardless of political affiliation. They emphasized the need for a peaceful transition of power in this time of uncertainty. These inspirational messages to the nation were being aired while former President Trump was in Florida. He left yesterday without participating in this event.

We have fallen from being the greatest country in the world by internal division. Together, we can rise from the ashes of this terrible pandemic, social inequities, and an unlawful insurrection. Only if we are united can we truly make America great again and move forward.

January 21, 2021

Today, I was working in the step-down unit, which is where folks go if they are too sick for the regular floor or not quite sick enough for the ICU. I was taking care of two patients who were brought from the jail with COVID. Guards have to escort those sick prisoners and stay with them in the room if they are admitted, ensuring they do not escape and the staff remain safe.

Every time I went in the guards were not wearing their protection. Although the guards are educated on how to put on the gown, gloves, face shield, and mask, in my experience, they rarely wear the gear. Maybe it's too difficult and would get in the way of reaching their weapon if that would be needed. But a mask and face shield? Now, guards are getting sick just like nurses in nursing homes. Nursing homes and jails are full of people in close quarters. Coronavirus spreads rampantly through those facilities, infecting residents and staff alike.

Most nurses are afraid of prisoners and don't like to talk to them much. I treat them just like regular folks and asked how they were feeling. Both of my prisoner patients had only one question—when they could get out of the hospital. Under normal circumstances they are happy for the change of pace and scenery.

"You guys are still really sick. You can't go back to the jail yet. Why are you so anxious to leave?" I asked one of the prisoners.

The younger one answered, "COVID at the jail is some scary shit. But you people walking around here in beekeeper space suits—that's freaking us out, man! This is like something in a bad movie where all the people die. I want outta here!"

I reassured him as best as I could. "We have to go above and beyond to protect ourselves because if we get sick then there would be nobody to take care of you."

Jan 22, 2021

Sandra called me to let me know her father was now in the hospital with low sodium and pneumonia. They were able to give him a new antibody combination drug called Regeneron. His primary diagnosis on admission was low sodium and not COVID. He does have COVID, and he was managing it at home by himself for that. He was not eating or drinking well, so it was really the low sodium that caused him to be admitted. If COVID was put as his primary diagnosis, the doctor said he wouldn't have been able to get the medication. Technically, it is only approved for outpatient use for COVID. It can be used if they are admitted to the hospital for something else, though. Who can understand that reasoning from the FDA or insurance companies?

January 23, 2021

Today was probably one of the strangest days of my entire career. When I arrived at work, I was designated as House Supervisor. The 'House Sup' generally oversees every department and all staff to ensure patients always get quality care. It is a big job, and I felt honored they considered me for this position. We had four critically ill patients who were not doing well. Their families put them on comfort care. Before my shift ended, I knew I would have to bag four bodies and take them to the overfilled morgue.

The weirdest thing happened next, which was the comic relief of the entire week. The chaplain passed by me walking in the hall and said, "Did you see the folks barbecuing outside of room four?"

I looked at him and gave a chuckle while I said, "You are funny, sir. That would be insane if it were true."

He looked back at me like a judge would stare down over his glasses at a defendant in court and said, "No, I would never joke about something like that."

We went to look out at the grassy courtyard. I knew he told me what was outside, but I could not even imagine what was in front of my eyes. There were about eight people hanging around one specific window, with fold-up chairs sitting by a bonafide functioning barbecue grill. The food was cooking, and people looked like they were having a party of a time. Can you imagine all those patients on BiPAP who have to choose to either eat or breathe, smelling that delicious aroma of mesquite lightly charred hamburgers and hot dogs? Or those patients who could eat, but didn't have family to bring them tasty treats like this from home? On top of that, I could not count all the rules they were breaking.

I found the security guard and asked her to come with me. She is this sweet, soft-spoken lady who wouldn't hurt a fly—but they didn't know that. I told her that I would be her muscle and would follow her lead. There is something about anyone in a uniform with the possibility of a weapon on their belt that makes people want to listen.

As we approached the family, I saw a husky guy carrying something heavy back out to the parking lot. There went the food. There were several people hanging out next to the window. An older lady was standing on one of the folding chairs trying to look in on the patient, rocking unsteadily back and forth on the uneven garden mulch. It looked like she was getting ready to fall to the ground and would then end up in the ER with a broken hip. She became startled once she saw me. Her legs started shaking as she tried to step down from the chair. I hurried to her side and reached out to help support her back down to safety.

The security guard apologized for breaking up their family reunion. She politely told them grilling was not permitted on hospital premises. Most of all, we couldn't allow family and friends looking through windows due to patient privacy laws, even if they knew their family member's room. After they walked away to the parking lot, the security guard and I looked at each other and busted out in hysterical laughter. I doubt I'll ever see anything like that again.

January 25, 2021

Most families across the US will be affected by this virus in some way before it's all over. I have a very large family, and everybody got together over the holidays. I'm sure nobody wore masks. When I heard my sister, a brother and his wife, and a niece tested positive, I lost my mind once again. I grew up in this little town where everyone knows most of the folks around them. This is a place where you think the virus would not likely raise its head. Unfortunately, this virus is very open to any location and any host. Nobody is safe.

My sister Charla tested positive for COVID and she lives with my momma. For a 79-year-old, my momma is in pretty good health, but she had some mild symptoms, too. She didn't want to leave the house, so she didn't get tested. I immediately called and told her to please not allow anyone in the house without a mask. Thankfully, they have not had to go to the hospital. Hopefully they will recover without further complications.

January 27, 2021

I wonder what our future will look like? Will it ever get back to "normal"? Will we need this vaccine like a yearly flu shot or just one every few years? It would be nice to see mask wearing become more widely accepted as a courtesy to others if someone was sick with even the common cold.

I saw on the news that the CDC changed the recommendation now to wear two cloth or surgical masks or one N95, as well as ten to twelve feet of social distance. They also announced a mask mandate on any public transportation or it is a federal offense.

The changes we are seeing in a response to this pandemic are not all bad. We have been forced to reinvent how we do business in order for this country's economy to survive. More people are working from home and most are being more productive.

In the early months of the crisis, we saw many layoffs in the hospitality industry that provide in-person service. As businesses began to change the way they function with take out or delivery options, some employees needed to be rehired. More online businesses required delivery personnel, which has helped unemployment. Increased ordering online from local stores and picking up items curbside has helped with sales, since there are limits on in-store occupancies.

This year has drastically changed our educational structure. Distance learning has a whole host of problems to consider. There is a lack of student engagement, whether it is an absence of desire, parental support, or sufficient space to learn. There is not equitable access to wifi, which crosses socio-economic lines. It is hard to provide different learning experiences for each student, especially those with special needs. There is also the insufficient contact to make personal connections between the students and teachers. How can our kids be successful in this handicapped learning environment?

How can we encourage our youth to get a secondary education when it is virtually cost prohibitive? In Colorado, in-state tuition for a state university is over $10,000 per year, without considering living expenses such as rent, food, car or public transportation, and don't forget about health insurance. How can a young person afford an education these days? A scientific major is labor intensive, and a part-time job may be impossible if one wants to keep a competitive grade point average. It would be great to have a national policy encouraging young people to go to college into a healthcare field by forgiving federal student loans. When another global health crisis arises, we will need to have sufficient essential workers trained and ready to go.

This year has drastically changed the face of healthcare. Many front-line workers were exposed early in this outbreak and thousands died. Healthcare workers of the large baby boomer generation are finding ways to consider early retirement after their experience in this pandemic. Some who are not old enough to retire are changing careers. They do not want to ever go through another pandemic again or anything even remotely like this. There were already not enough nurses going into nursing and not enough doctors going into medicine before this year.

I want to hug my momma and not worry about bringing her death by COVID. The only way I will be able to hug her safely is for most of the population in the world to get vaccinated, which is the only way to achieve herd immunity. This collective suffering with the COVID crisis will bring more PTSD than all twentieth century wars combined. Everyone will be affected, either directly or indirectly by this virus, before it's all over.

January 29, 2021

Kaitlyn called Sandra today to tell her she was sick with fever, headache, body aches, and felt awful. She went to the clinic and her test was negative. This presents a new dilemma. Our diagnostic tests detect genetic material or specific proteins from the virus. Researchers from Johns Hopkins have found the false negative rate is greater than one in five and sometimes is much higher. It takes time for the virus to replicate enough in the body to be detected. Having the test too early in the disease process may lead to a false negative result.

I have heard the nose swab test false negative rate is up to 30%. You may have the virus, but it might not be mainly in your nose or throat. The person doing the test may not have done it well enough. Some drive-thru testing sites ask the patient to do it themselves. I guarantee, most people won't shove that stick all the way up where it really needs to go. The test sample might not have been stored at the correct temperature while waiting for it to be processed.

The problem with false negative tests is that it gives the sick person the wrong impression they are not contagious, and it is not coronavirus. Then they go back to work or into society, spreading the infection. Kaitlyn did the responsible thing and quarantined in case she had COVID. We are watching and waiting now to see if Logan will get sick.

Lane and Dylton were finally recovered enough to be discharged today, but they are in such a weakened state, they cannot go home anytime soon. Dylton was transported to Hempstead, Texas to a rehab facility and was able to have the room next door to his wife. This was certainly a better situation for Lane to be close to her husband. She still couldn't see him because her coronavirus test remained positive, but they could talk through the door. Soon they both will be able to get the physical therapy needed to become strong enough to take care of themselves at home. I hope they reconsider permanently moving to the house close to Lane's daughters. They are in that time of life where assistance and close contact with adult children is important.

These days technology is so complicated, and changes are very fast. It is hard to keep up, especially when things are spiraling like in this crisis. New vaccines are coming out and it's important for me to stay up to date, no matter how busy I am.

There are different ways vaccines are made to work in the body. The first vaccines for COVID were the mRNA versions, which are very safe and have no virus pieces or parts. Other companies are looking into using a weak virus like adenovirus that causes the common cold to carry the genetic message to the cells to start making the spike protein. This is exactly like what the coronavirus would do to you. The spike protein then triggers an immune response to make antibodies. The good points about these adenovirus-based vaccines are the technology has been widely utilized in labs for a few decades. It is fast, well known, and cheap to use. The vaccine doesn't need a very cold fridge to be stored safely. The bad point is that since it has been around a long time, so many adults' immune systems already have specific antibodies to the adenovirus and would neutralize it. This is awful because we wouldn't know who in the community has neutralized the vaccine, so they will still be at risk.

Scientists are trying many different approaches to develop vaccines and not all of them will be successful for everyone. For example, some people are allergic to eggs, so they cannot take one type of vaccine. Another person has a weak immune system and can't take a live virus version. Variety in this technology is important to be able to cover as many people globally as possible.

January 31, 2021

The coronavirus outbreak affected every single individual on this entire planet in different ways from direct infection, affecting family and close friends, loss of jobs, or changing how we do our jobs, home schooling, mask wearing, social distancing, and the list goes on and on...

There were too many momentous issues we faced in 2020—fractured families, unemployment, divided communities, racial confrontations, political upheaval, catastrophic healthcare scenarios with COVID and numerous climate disasters. Even before the pandemic, many of these issues were inherently flawed. I would have thought an incredible global crisis like the one we are currently experiencing would have contributed to social cohesion, instead of dismantling what progress we have made.

A state of emergency uncovers the true character in people, from silent heroes to hidden villains—everyone is revealed. We see examples of both in our families, communities, and even on the national stage. Each and every one of us has a choice as to how we will respond in a crisis. If we decide to unite as one people in one nation with integrity, imagine what we could achieve. While there's no cure for the virus yet, I'm all in for chasing the cure to heal our nation. How about you?

	COVID CASES		COVID DEATHS	
JAN	Global 12,308	US 1	Global 265	US 0
FEB	Global 86,471	US 60	Global 2,978	US 0
MAR	Global 889,005	US 149,378	Global 45,236	US 5,210
APR	Global 3,482,232	US 1,086,625	Global 238,993	US 62,955
MAY	Global 6,515,313	US 1,856,560	Global 382,743	US 108,439
JUN	Global 10,575,194	US 2,762,809	Global 526,357	US 129,710
JUL	Global 17,627,792	US 4,708,945	Global 694,078	US 157,386
AUG	Global 26,012,690	US 6,234,482	Global 866,636	US 187,596
SEP	Global 34,891,132	US 7,532,411	Global 1,020,526	US 212,082
OCT	Global 47,161,108	US 9,395,274	Global 1,202,691	US 235,492
NOV	Global 63,485,398	US 13,998,001	Global 1,474,878	US 273,023
DEC	Global 83,943,230	US 20,502,143	Global 1,797,727	US 354,391
JAN	Global 103,116,285	US 26,658,053	Global 2,227,902	US 450,383

In the meantime, the numbers keep rising...

OTHER STORIES

In *Chasing the Surge* I told my personal story from my own experiences. I am one nurse. There are millions of other nurses, physicians, therapists, patients and families in the USA alone. Then there are all the millions of healthcare workers and patients in all the other countries in the world. They each have a similar and horrific story and yet unique to their own. Here are a few stories directly from some of those individuals and families who were affected by COVID.

CAMELIA'S STORY

I am a hospitalist and arrived to work in a small critical access hospital in rural Washington on March 18, 2020 for an eight day stretch. I felt a little run down as I had only two days off from my previous long shift.

I started having horrible low back pain, worse than anything I have felt before. Even the ED doc had no idea why I would suddenly experience this intense pain shooting down both legs. I was given some Flexeril as a muscle relaxer which worked minimally. I remember having to standing up leaning over the back of a recliner and actually fell asleep like that. I could not lie down in the bed because anything that touched the skin on my lower back would set me up on fire.

This went on for another three days. As the only physician admitting patients in a small, but busy hospital, I just pushed through knowing I had a ten day break coming up. I could make it 'til then. It really was miserable, but I was the only doc to care for these patients. I did not get much sleep between making rounds, night admissions from the ED, nursing phone calls, and sleeping like a horse standing up leaning over the lounge chair. I was exhausted.

I quickly started to get sick with fever and a dry cough which dropped into my chest and made me short of breath. I felt worse and worse by the hour with my knees shaking, weakness, and a gnawing feeling in the pit of my stomach telling me this was COVID.

At 11:00 p.m. the ED called me for another new admission. I realized right then I was incapable of caring for any patient in my condition. My fever was spiking. I told the ED doc I would be his next patient. I called the nurses and they came running. My temperature was 102.3, so they gave me Tylenol, and promptly loaded me onto a gurney to proceed to room #6 in the ED. I later learned the last patient in this same room came in with similar symptoms, worsened rapidly, and succumbed to COVID.

Now I was getting the hospital experience as a patient. I felt hopeless and scared. It certainly did not help when the staff came in to share their frightening coronavirus experiences with me. I see it from a different lens now. We medical professionals mean well. We always try to do our best, but when we talk between one another, we drop pretenses and decorum. Many times we use dark humor and bad language as tools to decompress, so we do not internalize every horror we see. We all do it. Sometimes aloud, sometimes in our minds. It is not meant to be disrespectful, but rather a buffer from the harshness of reality. At that point, I made a mental note as a physician to always be kind and on my best behavior with patients, and even when speaking to my colleagues.

When a physician becomes the patient, all the medical training goes out the window and the unexplainable, unwarranted, but real fears overwhelm all thoughts and reactions. I was waiting in room #6 for what seemed hours. I was so thirsty and had not eaten all day. I asked for water and it never came. I asked for crackers and it never came. At that moment, physically suffering and emotionally a wreck, I didn't care that everyone was busy. It was really frustrating. After all my years as a doctor, I can now empathize with patients who come to the hospital.

The ED doc came in and told me my temperature was better and my low blood pressure was responding to IV fluids, but my heart rate was 105 -110. My X-ray was not too bad, so the radiologist read it as normal. (Later we realized this report was incorrect due to the lack of knowledge with this new virus). My liver enzymes were high and I was bleeding like I was on blood thinners. I had numbness in my arms. Worst of all was the lack of taste and smell.

COVID had been in Washington for a little over a month and not much was known about this infection. And I had it. The ED doc told me how patients were rapidly progressing and being put on ventilators. When it got to that point, they were not likely to survive. Getting on a ventilator would be a death sentence for me. As a youth I was a smoker, sometimes a pack or more per day. Now I am proudly an ex-smoker, but I am sure damage was already done. I saw my father die of emphysema and I know that I can develop this later in life. I am overweight and not in the best cardiovascular shape, courtesy of a high stress job, low motivation to work out, and traveling many times a month from southern California to Washington State to work as a hospitalist in this little hospital.

And then something happened. I started to panic. I realized there was a possibility that I might not make it. I did not want to die in this small hospital in Washington state hundreds of miles away from my home. I have an eleven-year-old, a fourteen-year-old, and a husband I am missing terribly. I wanted to go home.

The news media was talking about the state shutting its borders in an effort to contain the pandemic. California was already infected in high numbers, and so was Oregon and Washington. I was supposed to take a flight home in two days, but here I was unable to stand up straight because my knees were buckling and I was coughing and with fever. I definitely could not get on that plane with this likely being COVID. But I could not stay here.

I was released with the promise that I would self-quarantine. I had a friend in Portland, Oregon with a small rental in the back of her house. Even though she was very scared of catching this infection, I was blessed she allowed me to stay. To this day, I have no idea how I successfully got in my rental car and made it there at her doorstep. She became my guardian angel bringing me food and necessary items to the door. I left my credit card out there as payment. We only communicated by text to not risk exposure to her or her daughters. I will always be with eternal gratitude to her for helping in my time of great need.

The following three to four days were a blur. I remember being in bed, then waking up in the middle of the night next to the toilet without any memory of getting there. I was vomiting, then heaving, and feeling miserable. Nothing tasted like anything. Water had a brash taste and I thought my cup was full of soap. I was so exhausted I could not even pick up the phone sitting on my chest and press the button to answer when it rang.

My colleagues were texting or calling me because they were fearful for my health and safety. I too was worried. I still believe to this day that I was closest to death with this illness than I have ever been in my life. Talking on the phone was beginning to be difficult as my oxygen level would drop to 81%. Looking in the mirror and seeing blue lips and purple fingers and toes did not help my situation. I started to think that I just might die in this vacation rental unit in Portland away from my beloved family. I started to cry which immediately triggered lung spasms and vomiting. It took a very long time afterward to catch my breath. I did not dare to check my oxygen level during all that.

I called my husband and told him I needed to come home. I was scared I would die without seeing my children again. Since I was speaking in full sentences at that moment, he did not take me seriously, of course. He should have heard me earlier in the morning when I was gurgling and gasping for breath. He did not see me when my temperature rose to over

104 nor when I passed out on the floor. Finally, he caught me at a time I could not say two consecutive words without coughing and gasping for air. He agreed to rent a van to have as much distance as possible between us and come get me. The drive home took thirty-five hours as my husband does not see well in low light. I was forced to take the driver's seat. I placed a pillow on the wheel to support my chest. As long as I did not move too much, I was okay. Getting up and down and definitely walking to the bathroom took so much effort and turned me blue and purple again. My cough was relentless, my muscles were aching, and food was unpalatable. I felt like I was in hell. Somehow, we made it home.

The following days would have been comical, if I had felt better to enjoy it. The dog was constantly scratching at my quarantined bedroom door and whining wanting to come in. He even serenaded me with a few howls of painful indignation, not knowing why I wouldn't let him enter. I remember my son bringing my breakfast. He had his chemistry goggles on, a huge hat, sunglasses, three masks, and gloves too big for his hands and huge overalls. He rushed in with the tray spilling water and coffee as he was holding his breath trying his hardest to get the hell out of there as fast as possible. Then I heard the cleaning spray hissing on the outside doorknob and down the stairwell. I smiled knowing that at least they were being smart enough to sanitize behind them.

I reached my worst point at the beginning of April. I remember 4:00 in the morning feeling exhausted, hearing my lungs gurgling, unable to take deep breaths, unable to oxygenate. Shaking and fearful, I decided it was time to go the hospital. I knew that with my oxygen in the 70s and my vision getting blurry, I could not avoid intubation. I was dizzy from the lack of oxygen and did not feel good.

But like every good girl who listens to her momma, I had to make sure I had a clean pair of knickers on me when I go to the doctor. So, I dragged myself in the shower trying to get clean before I called my husband to take me to the ER. I could not stand, so I was lying on the tile floor, but the hot water and steam made it really hard to breathe. I started coughing so viciously, ripping in my chest that I thought my lung tissue was tearing loose. Then I felt something pop and an alien looking thing came out of my mouth. It looked like a yellowish waxy cast of a lung branch. I realized that this is what we in medicine call a mucous plug that was obstructing my airway that I was able to dislodge to breathe again. My impending doom vanished. That was finally my turning point and I started getting better from there.

I realized that moist heat actually helped induce a deeper cough. I also realized that having my husband pound on my back also helped loosen the secretions. I used our sports massager to vibrate my back as a chest percussion therapy device every morning and night to help me get rid of all this bloody mucous. My heart was still beating fast about 120-130. This is consistent with inflammation around the heart called pericarditis. But now I was getting better by leaps and bounds.

On April 7 I went outside in the backyard for twenty minutes. I looked up to the sun and felt the warmth on my face, heard the hummingbirds zooming around, the insects making noise in the flowers. It felt so good, so new, so refreshing, like a new lease on life. Everything was bright, green blades of grass, the reds of the flower pedals in the flower bed. I could hear the munching of my tortoise that was grazing on the grass at my feet and it was delightful. I enjoyed nature like a small child and was so grateful to be alive.

I realized that my children did not grasp how close I was to death as I was isolated upstairs in my room. My daughter told me, "I cried so hard when you told me you wanted to see me one more time before you died. Then Khonsura (her step-dad) told me you were just exaggerating and were just fine, so I stopped being scared." My son was a proud Republican at the young age of fourteen (to the rest of the household consternation, as we are all Democrats). He bought into all of the fake news and conspiracy of the 'China virus' that was only going to ruin his social life. He did not think I was actually diagnosed with COVID.

It is amazing how even with all the proof in front of their noses some people cannot and will not admit to something they cannot understand. My own children saw me so sick for weeks, turning blue, heard me practically coughing up what looked like a lung and believed this was just another virus, and not a big deal.

Just as a disclosure, now I realize how I got sick. My daughter got sick at school with the sniffles for two or three days. My step-son was sick with muscle aches and lost taste for about a week and my husband was ill, all of them just before me in March. Looking back, I am certain they all had COVID and none of us realized it.

I was off work until June and really needed all that time to recuperate and renew mentally and physically. I am back to work and doing my job well, feeling confident as ever. I am working harder than ever. But even now almost a year later, I am still having lasting effects of this infection. I definitely have COVID brain. I am not losing my keys or forgetting my kid's names, but I find rote memorization hard to do now. I don't feel as sharp as I was before I got sick. My lungs are not the same either. I cannot speak a long sentence without having to stop in the middle to catch my breath. I cannot run up the stairs at home without feeling winded. I have insomnia. If I have a fever or a body ache, I get those panic attacks that make me hyperventilate. I know this is PTSD.

Have you ever felt close to death? Have you ever felt that you cannot breathe like having a plastic bag tied tight over your head? Have you ever felt like you were going to have a heart attack because your heart was beating so fast that it was physically hurting you? Now if I feel anything out of the ordinary, I relive those memories and that anxious feeling comes flooding back. It is terrifying.

Even though I was scared to return to the hospital where this all started, I could not financially stay home anymore. I also swore an oath both to serve and heal my fellowman. I have to uphold my end of the bargain no matter the risk.

I realize now why doctors and nurses volunteered to go to New York risking their lives and several of them died. They all have that sense of duty that I have. When you become a doctor or nurse, your life is not your own anymore. Your wellbeing is important, but your patient's needs supersede yours any day.

Keeping a patient alive is a privilege. Helping a person heal allowing them to go back to their family is such a blessing. On the other hand, I have pronounced more people dead in this COVID pandemic in nine months than in my entire medical career combined. When multiple patients were all deteriorating at once and dying one after the other, I felt worthless as a doctor. I felt it was my fault. We were walking around crying and feeling hopeless. We could not transfer them to a larger hospital as nobody had any room.

The positive aspect to this was that the medical community grew closer as we all were fighting a common enemy. Strangers on the other end of the phone were so willing to share their experience and give helpful advice at any time of the day or night. I see all around me in this country and across the world what we humans are able to do when we are joined by selflessness and a common goal. When we put our minds and hearts together and egos aside, humanity as a collective can reach the stars. We can overcome anything that we put our minds to do. We can heal ourselves and this planet. We can leave a legacy of good will and peace behind...or we can continue to march the same way to our peril. That is our choice. I hope we all have learned compassion with the many deaths in this pandemic and I hope it has given us wisdom for the future.

MAXINE'S STORY

Robert Wayne Elliot was my brother and my best friend. We grew up in the back country of Tennessee with eight siblings. When we were little, we found it hard to say "Robert Wayne", so I've only known him as "Wot Wayne."

Our family has a history of kidney disease and high blood pressure. Robert was not spared. He had been on dialysis for a while. Doctors were trying to get him a transplant soon. Because of his medical issues, he was very careful since the beginning of this pandemic.

Robert Wayne lived in a senior citizen apartment building on the second floor. He never went anywhere, except to dialysis. Three times a week he walked down the stairs to catch the bus to go to his treatments. Otherwise, he never left his apartment.

On Wednesday after New Year, he started feeling weaker than usual. He went to his normal dialysis treatment, but they could not treat him. He had a high fever. They called an ambulance which took him straight to the hospital. He was diagnosed with COVID and admitted in the hospital.

He struggled with fever, aches and pains, but did not end up in the ICU like some other people we know. I work in the hospital cafeteria, so I know how bad this can get. My nephew's wife is a physician assistant. She also works at the hospital. With her help, I was lucky to see my brother during those weeks he was in treatment. So many other families never get to see their loved ones ever again, I know this is true.

Robert was in the hospital for over two and a half weeks. He was so weak after getting COVID, he could barely walk. He couldn't go home because there was no way he could go up and down all those stairs. The doctors got him into rehab for physical therapy. He got better. After a week in therapy, Wayne started coughing up blood, and was sent right back to the hospital. The doctors had to transfuse him to get his blood count up, then got him dialysis.

One night after he had been in the hospital another week, he was feeling better. He was getting ready to go back to rehab. My niece FaceTimed with him. We all told him how we miss and love him.

Wot Wayne said he was happy and feeling good about going back to rehab for therapy. We spoke about him coming to live with me instead of going back to his apartment. He was excited about that and said, "I beat the COVID and gonna go live with my sister! What else could I ask for?" It was such a long month for him. I was glad to see him finally sounding more like his old self.

The next morning my sister called and asked if I had heard about Robert. He had a massive heart attack last night and died on January 31.

After my brother's death, we figured out how he probably got COVID. He became sick on Wednesday, January 6. His neighbor lady downstairs died of COVID the next day, January 7. They did not visit at all, so he was not directly exposed to her. We suspect the air vents in the building was the way this disease got to my brother.

We still do not have a death certificate. There have been so many deaths that mortuaries are backlogged. We are number forty in the line to get our brother cremated. Then, we can have his funeral and finally have closure.

There have been a lot of other deaths after Robert. I can't imagine where in this small town they are keeping all the bodies that need to be buried. I am sure this is a big problem everywhere, but we don't hear about this on the news. This waiting has made us have a lot of questions about why this had to happen in the first place. Our family with ten kids now has only four. We are sad and grieving our loss. We are extremely angry. Robert's death could have been avoided.

If our government would have just listened to the experts and warned us sooner, hundreds of thousands of people could have been spared; people just like my brother. Their families are in the same place as me. Are they angry at how all this happened? Are they still not able to have closure like us? Robert would want us to move on and be happy. It will take a very long time for us to get to a better place to be able to forgive, and never can we forget.

We love you and miss you lots, Wot Wayne; my brother; my best friend.

—Maxine Elliot

FRED'S STORY

My dad, Fred, is an 84-year-old retired farmer from California. His parents immigrated from Germany and Switzerland in 1929. Their family established the first dairy farm in Oregon, White Rose Dairy. Fred grew up milking cows and working hard sunup to sundown delivering milk to customers. He vowed he would never be a dairyman when he grew up.

Fred put himself through school by working construction jobs in the summers. He was then able to concentrate on his studies and graduated from Oregon State University with a double major in Engineering and Business. He also played football in school and was an avid snow and water skier, Mt Hood in the winter and the Columbia River in the summer.

I am telling you all this about his past so you can really see what type of man he is and this story I am about to tell you did not happen to the weak. In the early 70s, Fred went into full-time farming and became one of the largest potato producers in California. I remember early on when we first were getting started, we had to clear the land of all the rocks before we could work the soil. I was so proud that he let me drive the Model M tractor while my dad and mom loaded all the rocks on the trailer. Our family focus was to work hard and play hard...together.

We grew potatoes, onions, grain, and garlic. As a young girl I helped a lot on the farm. Work responsibilities always took precedence over any personal agenda. I remember the competition in tallying the number of rows of irrigation pipe laid in a day or rows cultivated by each of the crew. At lunch, we compared what we were able to get done so far, never minding the condiment of dirt from our hands on our sandwiches.

My dad was always strong and capable. Even after he got older, he remained very active, more so than most men his age. He still enjoyed golfing, snow skiing. and water skiing.

Fred and Jessie are the proverbial snowbirds. They live six months in Klamath Falls and 'fly south' to Arizona for the winter. This year, Thanksgiving was going to be nice. The plan was for me and my husband and our three adult kids and all the significant others to travel down from Fallon, Nevada to Wickenburg, Arizona to spend the holiday weekend with my folks.

During this COVID pandemic Fred and Jessie listened to the news reports and did everything they could to stay protected. They took all the recommended precautions against exposures and limited their social life to a small group of friends and family.

Fred's COVID experience began in November 2020 when he and Jessie returned to Arizona as was usual this time of year. The two-day travel from Klamath Falls was exhausting. On the road, they could not stop to eat anywhere as the restaurants were take-out only due to COVID. They stopped in Coalinga, California to sleep in a hotel and was met with a very limited room service menu...a bowl of soup for dinner.

Continuing on the road the next day, Fred actually fell asleep at the wheel. This could have been a disaster but for the Lane Change Alert on their Audi, they remained unscathed without an accident or injury. The tired couple arrived in Wickenburg on November 19 to settle in for the winter and holiday season. They knew Cindy was coming with the troops the next week to cook and visit.

Thanksgiving week was not at all what they had planned. On Sunday before Thanksgiving, my dad started having extreme shakes of both his arms and legs. He went to the ED and was diagnosed with COVID. He spent three days in the hospital leaving his wife Jessie at home alone.

I live in Fallon, Nevada but needed to step up and care for my parents as they struggled with this time of illness. It would likely be just a few weeks and I could work from there without a problem. I got to Arizona just in time to bring Dad home from his first stay in the hospital. He was home only three days when again his oxygen started dropping to 85% and I took him back to the ED. I knew it would be several hours of tests and an examination, so I went back to the house to be with my mom.

As I arrived home, I walked into the door and was met with the most awful smell of vomit and feces. My mother had projectile vomiting and watery diarrhea all over the place! It was all I could do to keep from gagging. I found her in the powder room in a heavy sweat mumbling incoherently. I called 911 and proceeded to get her cleaned up for her trip to the hospital.

As the couple sat across from each other in the emergency department, I overheard their conversation,

"What in the hell are you doing here?" Fred asked his wife.

"It's a long story," she replied, as he was wheeled to his room.

Jessie was treated with IV fluids and diarrhea medications, then released while Fred was placed in Observation. This second hospital stay was less than two days and he was discharged again back into my care on Christmas Eve.

These weeks turned into months as this COVID saga continued to unfold. On December 30, Dad had an appointment with his PCP. During my entire life, my father was the strong and capable type, not needing much help to do anything. Having COVID completely decimated his strength that we had so much difficulty getting him in and out of the car and to the office door. We were fifteen minutes late to the appointment and were turned away. They did not understand how deteriorated he was and at risk for needing to be readmitted to the hospital. We needed him to be seen by his doctor but that just was not going to happen today. The staff were operating according to their protocol and unwilling to bend.

I brought Dad home after an exhausting afternoon, finally got him settled in his chair, and took his vitals. Blood pressure 198/96 with oxygen 87%. Once again, we went to the ED, got him registered and I drove away feeling the helplessness of this revolving door. Six hours later at 1:00 a.m., the call came that he did have low oxygen and with severe anemia, but he did not meet criteria for admission. He needed to come home.

The next morning, I left the house for about thirty minutes to go to the pharmacy down the street to pick up some prescriptions for my mom and dad. As I walked back in the house, carrying all the bags of medicines and other items, chatting away as I usually do, there was no response from Fred. He was sitting at the computer facing the window with his back turned to me. I assumed he was searching the internet or reading an email. "Dad?" I called. "Dad!" I dropped the bags and rushed to him, shaking him with no response other than unintelligible sounds. I called a physician friend and explained all that was going on. Of course, the only thing to do was to call 911. Yet again.

This time, the EMTs on arrival decided to bypass the local hospital and fly him by helicopter to the larger hospital in Phoenix. Thankfully, I have contacts in that hospital system due to my job and was able to communicate directly with the ED provider giving all the recent complicated history since November.

He was admitted for the third time on December 31 to the ICU. Then in the middle of the night they needed the ICU bed for someone in worse shape. He was moved to a COVID ward that had been set up in an old unoccupied wing of the hospital. His diagnosis...Acute Stroke.

Here is where the story gets crazy. Remember, my father is 84-years-old and now has been reduced to an incapacitated level of weakness. He cannot care for himself at all. His new room in this isolated unit was very small for one person, but there were two patients sharing it. His roommate who also was COVID-positive, had severe uncontrollable watery diarrhea from this infection. The roommate continuously soiled the floor on the way to the bathroom many times every hour with the stench of feces constantly permeating the air, even at mealtimes.

The nurses were stressed and overworked, but still came into the room at all times of the day and night, not letting the patients sleep. Dad remembers being able to sleep typically between 11p.m. and 1a.m., but his perception was that this was actually in the afternoon. He was confused and not getting better. After the seventh day, he finally seemed to be more alert. He was able to tell me that there had been no heat in that section of the hospital and his room was 55 degrees! He was freezing! It turned out that nobody knew how to adjust the thermostat! Finally, after twenty days in that misery, plans were being made to get him to rehab before coming back home. But his hospital stay was not yet over.

The one luxury he longed for was to shave his beard. He hated to be scruffy. My brothers were able to drop off a razor at the front desk which was delivered to him so he could groom himself. Unfortunately, the staff were so taxed that he never got help with a shave and not once did he get a shower during this twenty-day admission.

The conditions were certainly awful in the hospital, but there were several tender moments of humanity shared between my dad and the nurses. He had horrible urine incontinence likely from the stroke and was constantly wetting his clothes and the bed. After multiple failed attempts to place a catheter, the nurse came in sheepishly with the hospital version of an adult diaper for him to have some dignity. They had a little laugh over this, and the humor was very welcome.

Dad always treated people with respect and even in his time of suffering, he understood what they were doing and the sacrifices they were making to care for those with this virus. The respect was returned by the majority. When the food provided was inedible, the nurses would bring him pudding with graham crackers and milk. Although not very nutritious, it did help satiate the need for comfort foods and encourage restfulness.

He was finally discharged on January 18 to the Acute Rehab which felt like the Taj Mahal after the last twenty days in that makeshift COVID unit. We were able to drop off personal items to make his stay more comfortable, but still could not make any contact. He had not seen his family since he was taken from the house in the ambulance to the helicopter on December 31.

Being an administrator in a physician led company, I understood the process in hospitals and was able to navigate the numerous roadblocks to getting information. I was able to connect with the nursing staff, Case Managers, and physicians regarding the state of my father's health and his slow recovery. Without my professional experience, there would have been little to no communication with the immediate or extended family.

He finally came home from rehab on his birthday, January 20. What a celebration! But we were completely unprepared to address his limited mobility. I made numerous trips to the pharmacy for shower seats, shower matts, grab bars that needed to be installed, walkers (one regular one and one with the seat), handheld shower head also needing installation, heating pads, and a lift chair recliner as he could not get up unassisted.

My brother Mike and I alternated so that Fred and Jessie would have someone with them 24/7 and we could each have time to recuperate in our respective homes periodically. We were away from our families, but it is what we as adult children need to do. It is very hard to be thrown abruptly into the role of immediate full-time caregivers as we have our family and personal needs that had to take a back seat for now. Our professional careers cannot be put on hold, so we learned quickly how to multitask to an exponential degree.

This horrific experience comes with a happy ending. Upon discharge from Acute Rehab, Dad's progress had been slow, but steady. After two weeks (February 21, 2021), he was able to walk without a walker, and most recently took a trip down to the driving range to chip and putt. He still is having weak spells in his legs and took a fall that required two of us to get him up. Yet, I am encouraged each day we get farther from his COVID nightmare. Dad is able to do more and more for himself eventually gaining back his independence.

We are grateful to still have my father with us as there are millions of families that were not so fortunate and grieving the loss of their loved ones.

KOURTNEE'S STORY

My dad's memory will not be lost in vain. It took sixteen days from receiving a positive COVID-19 result to his last breath. As an employee of our critical access hospital, I've been mask fitted, trained in proper PPE wear, certified on COVID patient contact, and vaccinated with the Pfizer COVID-19 vaccine. Since I was an employee, I had access to my father as a patient. It was a surreal chapter of my life.

I felt helpless watching my dad's health decline for sixteen days. Every day he became worse. As I watched him struggle more and more, the nonstop scenarios ran through my mind. I knew what could happen to the most beloved man in my life.

On January 9, 2021 my dad Stephen, was rushed to the emergency room for the third time that week. ICU orders were placed within half an hour of being registered. He was placed on a BIPAP machine within hours of arrival. He slept non-stop, wouldn't eat a bite, didn't have energy to open his eyes, let alone speak, and remained septic.

He could not get into a proper ICU room for another eight days. I felt torn feeling lucky enough to be present with my dad, but also full of heartache and inevitability because of his critical condition.

On January 14, 2021 at 1:00 in the morning I received a call which woke me up. It was a nursing staff member from the ICU department requesting permission to intubate my dad. His vitals were not maintaining, so this was a last resort. I gave permission without hesitation. I sobbed by myself at home in bed. In the black of night, I cried harder than I had ever cried before.

As an employee who works in the emergency department and within the hospital, I have physically seen the process of intubation. I spoke with physicians and nursing staff about patient intubation, ventilators and life expectancy prior to my dad ever contracting coronavirus. I knew the grim outcome. It hurt beyond belief to know my once strong, independent, loving, playful, hardworking, and smart-mouthed father was experiencing such a tragic ending.

Wednesday, January 20, 2021 while working, I received a call from the ICU department advising me that my dad was no longer maintaining health and was rapidly declining. The two previous days were rough. He had uncontrollable fever, high blood sugar, a urinary tract infection, up and down respiratory and oxygen levels, and more. His blood pressure dropped so low even four rounds of medication would not bring it up, and it only continued to drop.

Staff requested my mother to be brought in to see her husband for her final goodbye. It was the most painful call that I've ever received. Then I had to make another most painful call within a few minutes. Once my mother and two of my sisters arrived, we fully gowned and covered up to enter his ICU room. As a family we released my dad from two sedation medications, blood pressure medications, and then the ventilator.

He had three of his five daughters surrounding him, along with his loyal wife Susan. We assured our unconscious dad we loved him and were present with him. We explained we were going to be okay and we were selflessly letting go. Our hearts ache and we mourn for the most important and influential man we lost in sixteen short days. We have yet to fully feel the effects of his absence, and we miss him beyond words.

At the same time, I am extremely grateful to have been able to see my dad daily for his last sixteen days. This is a privilege no other family member has now. I was blessed to be able to enter his room, read to him, comb his hair, and tell him about my day and about his own condition. I was honored to be able to touch his skin and face and hold his hand. Since I personally knew and worked beside the staff who cared for him, I was kept up to date with every step and issue or improvement he experienced. Most importantly, I was able to reassure my dad that it was okay to let go when he was ready. Honoring my dad's wishes and releasing him from artificial life was both cathartic and heart breaking. I knew I would lose my best friend, caring dad, loving husband to Susan, and overall fun spirited, passionate-about-life kind of man, and none of us could bear to see him suffer any more.

My family mourns his death. We also crusade for a safer world, a healthier world, and a united world by practicing social distancing, mask wearing, hand cleansing, along with education and prevention. If this experience and pain filled loss can help just one family prevent a death, then my dad's legacy is important. The virus and contagion is real; it does not discriminate nor does it hold back.

— Kourtnee Jackson

DARDEN'S STORY

In early January I called my friend Tom to talk about an upcoming project. When I asked him how he was doing he said he wasn't doing so well, as his wife Lynn had been in the hospital for a month with COVID-19. She had been on a respirator, then off, but was now back on it. I'm not a doctor, but I knew that wasn't a good sign. As Tom and I talked, he got more emotional. He told me that he and Lynne met when they were fifteen, and had been married for forty years, that she was his everything, his best friend. At several points in the conversation, he broke down. At one point he said, "I know there's nothing you can do, but you're the one that called, so you get to listen to me."

I hesitated for a moment, and said, "Well, there is one thing I can do."

"What's that?"

"It might sound strange, but we can write a song for Lynne." I answered.

"How?" Tom asked.

"You talk, I'll write it down. Together we can write it and get the song to Lynne."

Tom laughed and said, "Bud, she's in a coma."

"Tom, I can record it, we send an mp3 to the nurses. They can put headphones on Lynne and play it for her. And I guarantee that if we write exactly what you feel, Lynne will hear the song and know it's your words. She'll hear it. Don't worry."

I've been writing songs since I was ten. It's my way of moving through the world. Along with writing for my own recording projects, around twenty years ago I became fascinated with developing songs with people who don't write songs, helping them tell their stories in a new way. I've done work with homeless teenagers, gangs, conflict resolution work with Israeli/Palestinian groups, companies and couples. I co-founded an organization called Songwriting With Soldiers, where we paired professional songwriters with veterans to turn their stories of combat and the return home into songs.

Songs are truth bombs. They connect the writer and the singer and the listener like no other medium. They can turn the darkest, saddest story into a thing of beauty that people will sing with joy. I knew this would work.

I asked Tom to just tell me how he felt about Lynne. What was their love like?

He said, "She is my best friend. It's forever. It really is true love."

I said, "Forever true." He started to cry. I knew we had our title.

After a while it became difficult for Tom to keep talking, so I suggested he think about it and text me throughout the day with anything about Lynne or their life together that came to mind. From the words in his texts, and the things I'd written down during our conversation, I was able to put together a rough sketch of the song.

Later that evening, something told me that I needed to go back up to the studio and finish the recording. I had a feeling that I didn't have much time. It took about another hour to finish and send it to Tom. He immediately forwarded a copy to the nurses, who played Lynne her song.

The following day Tom told me that after the nurses played *Forever True* for Lynne, her vitals changed a bit for the better. She improved during the day. Was it the song? I can't say. I believe that it was the spirit of it—the collaboration of Tom and I, along with the nurses to bring a little light to Lynne. She somehow knew what was going on.

Unfortunately Lynne died several days later. Tom and I are forever bonded, and he now has a memorial to his love for Lynne. He was able to speak his truth, and I believe Lynne heard her song, and responded. The next week, I played the song in a livestream concert. It was requested for weeks in my shows. People asked for copies of the lyrics. I'm touched to find how I can help people who cannot have contact, connect during their most critical time in this personal way.

The COVID crisis hit home for me when I heard Grover discuss his experiences on an interview. I felt compelled to reach out to him to see if he would be interested in writing a song with me about his experiences and challenges over this past year. It was cathartic for both of us. His song is a call for us to come together in unity for everything, not just the fight against COVID, but to heal the other issues dividing our country.

We all have the ability to make a difference in our own unique way. I write songs, so that's what I give to the world. The best way for us to make a difference is to do what we're best at, to use our strengths for good, and to serve others by being ourselves.

FOREVER TRUE

Darden Smith / Tom Burns

With a heart so full of wonder
And the light upon your face
Eyes that spark like diamonds
A soul so full of grace
All of our tomorrows
And all those yesterdays

Forever and ever
I'll be loving you
Forever, forever true

Though the years might run like water
Though the tears might fall like rain
The love and all the laughter
That's that will remain
In every waking moment
Inside every dream

© 2021 Darden Smith Music (ASCAP)

TOGETHER

Grover Nicodemus Street / Darden Smith

Late night headlights my life goes by
A year's worth of tears filling up my eyes
For those that lived and breathe with grace
For those that passed to another place
I did all that I could do
And I'd do it all again for you

We the people got to come together
Serve each other, make the world better
See the beauty of the soul and not the color of skin
Find that love that's deep within
Arm and arm hand and hand
Stand together

Real life scary movie, a never-ending dream
I swam in the ocean of COVID-19
While some tried to hide, turn their eyes away
I've been down to the bottom but I'm here today
Reaching out to the other side
Calling out across the great divide

We the people got to come together
Serve each other, make the world better
See the beauty of the soul and not the color of skin
Find that love that's deep within
Arm and arm hand and hand
Stand together

I've seen beauty in the face of pain
I've seen faith in time of tear
When we go beyond, we go above

The fear that's always here

We the people can come together
Serve one another make the whole world better
See the beauty of soul and not the color of the skin
Sing the song of love calling deep within
Arm and arm hand and hand
Stand together
Come together

@ Frontline Songs (BMI) / Darden Smith Music (ASCAP)

SOURCES

Alter, Charlotte. "Black Lives Matter Protest in New York Attracts New People." *Time,* 10 July 2016, https://time.com/4400211/black-lives-matter-new-york-protest/. Accessed 2021.

Anglesey, Anders. "Fact Check: Did George Floyd Die of a Drug Overdose, as Tucker Carlson Says?" *Newsweek,* 11 Feb. 2021, https://www.newsweek.com/fact-check-george-floyd-cause-death-1568687. Accessed 2021.

Anguiano, Dani. "California's wildfire hell: how 2020 became the state's worst ever fire season." *The Guardian,* 30 Dec. 2020, https://www.theguardian.com/us-news/2020/dec/30/california-wildfires-north-complex-record. Accessed 2021.

Associated Press. "75-year-old protester shoved to ground by Buffalo police has skull fracture: lawyer." *Cbc.ca.* Canadian Broadcasting Corporation, 17 June 2020. Web. Accessed 2021.

Associated Press. "Officers suspended after shoving 75-year-old to the ground, cracking his skull." *Politico,* 5 July 2020, https://www.politico.com/news/2020/06/05/buffalo-police-new-york-city-protests-303168. Accessed 2021.

COVID-19 Treatment Guidelines Panel. Coronavirus Disease 2019 (COVID-19) Treatment Guidelines. National Institutes of Health. Available

At https://www.covid19treatmentguidelines.nih.gov/. Accessed 2021.

Crump, Andy, and Satoshi Ōmura. "Ivermectin, 'wonder drug' from Japan: the human use perspective." *Proceedings of the*

Sources

Japan Academy. Series B, Physical and biological sciences vol. 87,2 (2011): 13-28. doi:10.2183/pjab.87.13

"Derek Chauvin." *Wikipedia,* Wikimedia Foundation, 23 March 2021, https://en.wikipedia.org/w/index.php?title=Derek_Chauvin&action=history.

"Dr. Fauci on coronavirus fears: No need to change lifestyle yet." *USA Today,* 29 Feb. 2020, https://www.today.com/video/dr-fauci-on-coronavirus-fears-no-need-to-change-lifestyle-yet-79684677616. Accessed 2021.

"Eight minutes 46 seconds." *Wikipedia,* Wikimedia Foundation, 22 March 2021, https://en.wikipedia.org/wiki/Eight_minutes_46_seconds.

FDA Approves First Treatment for COVID-19. U.S. Food & Drug Administration, 22 Oct. 2020, https://www.fda.gov/news-events/press-announcements/fda-approves-first-treatment-covid-19#:~:text=Veklury%20is%20the%20first%20treatment,to%20receive%20FDA%20approval. Accessed 2021.

FPJ Web Desk. "'He fell harder than he was pushed': Trump wonders if old man whose skull cracked open in Buffalo was a 'set up'." *The Free Press Journal,* 9 June 2020, https://www.freepressjournal.in/world/he-fell-harder-than-he-was-pushed-trump-wonders-if-old-man-whose-skull-cracked-open-in-buffalo-was-a-set-up. Accessed 2021.

"George Floyd protests in New York City." Wikipedia, Wikimedia Foundation, 15 Feb. 2021. https://en.wikipedia.org/w/index.php?title=George_Floyd_protests_in_New_York_City&action=history.

"George Floyd protests." *Wikipedia,* Wikimedia Foundation, 21 March 2021, https://en.wikipedia.org/w/index.php?title=George_Floyd_protests&action=history.

Golden, Hallie. "Seattle protestors take over city blocks to create police-free 'autonomous zone'." *The Guardian,* 11 Jun. 2020, https://www.theguardian.com/us-news/2020/jun/11/chaz-seattle-autonomous-zone-police-protest. Accessed 2021.

Hahn, Stephen. "Oversight of the Administration's Response to the COVID-19 Pandemic." *U.S. Food and Drug Administration,* 23 June 2020, www.fda.gov/news-events/congressional-testimony/oversight-trump-administrations-response-covid-19-pandemic-06232020. Accessed 2021.

Hoft, Jim. "Breaking: HHS Secretary Alex Azar Announces FDA Authorized Coronavirus Vaccine to Enter Phase One Testing." *Thegatewaypundit.com.* Gateway Pundit, 2020, https://www.thegatewaypundit.com/2020/03/breaking-hhs-secretary-alex-azar-announces-fda-authorized-coronavirus-vaccine-to-enter-phase-one-testing-video/. Accessed 2021.

Kimball, Spencer. "'We're built up with frustration': Scenes and sounds in NYC during 3 days of protests against police brutality." *cnbc.com.* NBCUniversal News Group, 6 June 2020. Web. Accessed 2021.

Lee, Jessica. "Background Check: Investigating George Floyd's Criminal Record." *Snopes,* Snopes Media Group, 12 June 2020, https://www.snopes.com/news/2020/06/12/george-floyd-criminal-record/. Accessed 2021.

Sources

Leichman, Abigail. "Israelis testing anti-parasite drug against Covid-19: Sheba Medical Center specialist begins clinical trial of ivermectin, hoping it could shorten the duration of the infection to a few days." *ISRAEL21c,* 16 June 2020, https://www.israel21c.org/israelis-testing-anti-parasite-drug-against-covid-19/. Accessed 2021.

Lewis, Sophie. "California wildfires have already burned 2.2 million acres in 2020- more than any year on record." *Cbsnews.com*. CBS NEWS, 9 Sept. 2020. Web. Accessed 2021

McCausland, Phil. "CDC warns against using form of chloroquine that killed man, sickened his wife." *Nbcnews.com.* NBC News, 28 Mar. 2020. Web. Accessed 2021.

Mega, Emiliano. "Latin America's embrace of an unproven COVID treatment is hindering drug trials." *Nature, vol.* 586, 22 Oct. 2020, pp.481-482, https://www.nature.com/articles/d41586-020-02958-2. Accessed 2021.

Musto, Julia. "HHS Secretary Alex Azar encouraged by proposed coronavirus vaccine timeline." *Foxnews.com.* Fox News Network, 4 March 2020. Web. Accessed 2021.

Neuman, Scott. "Man Dies, Woman Hospitalized After Taking Form of Chloroquine to Prevent COVID-19." *Npr.com,* npr, 24 Mar. 2020, https://www.npr.org/sections/coronavirus-live-updates/2020/03/24/820512107/man-dies-woman-hospitalized-after-taking-form-of-chloroquine-to-prevent-covid-19. Accessed 2021.

Neuman, Scott. "Medical Examiner's Autopsy Reveals George Floyd Had Positive Test For Coronavirus." *npr.com,* npr, 4 June

2020, https://www.npr.org/sections/live-updates-protests-for-racial-justice/2020/06/04/869278494/medical-examiners-autopsy-reveals-george-floyd-had-positive-test-for-coronavirus. Accessed 2021.

O'Donnell, Jayne. "Top disease official: Risk of coronavirus in USA in 'miniscule'; skip mask and wash hands." *USA TODAY,* 17 Feb. 2020, https://www.usatoday.com/story/news/health/2020/02/17/nih-disease-official-anthony-fauci-risk-of-coronavirus-in-u-s-is-minuscule-skip-mask-and-wash-hands/4787209002/. Accessed 2021.

Perez, Matt. "Trump Suggests Injecting Coronavirus Patients with Light Or Disinfectants, Alarming Experts." *Forbes,* 24 Apr. 2020, https://www.forbes.com/sites/mattperez/2020/04/23/trump-suggests-injecting-coronavirus-patients-with-light-or-disinfectants-contradicting-experts/?sh=72de332a4088. Accessed 2021.

Phillips, Amber. "3 Takeaways from Thursday's White House coronavirus briefing." *The Washington Post,* 23 Apr. 2020, https://www.washingtonpost.com/politics/2020/04/23/white-house-coronaivrus-briefing-takeaways/. Accessed 2021.

"President Trump with Coronavirus Task Force Briefing." *C-SPAN,* uploaded by C-SPAN, 23 Apr. 2020, https://www.c-span.org/video/?471458-1/president-trump-coronavirus-task-force-briefing.

Public Citizen. "Top Ways Trump Sped Up the Spread of Coronavirus." *Top 12 Things Trump Did to Speed the Pandemic,* Public Citizen, 27 May 2020, https://www.citizen.org/news/

top-12-things-trump-did-to-speed-the-pandemic/. Accessed 2021.

"Rosa Parks." *Wikipedia,* Wikimedia Foundation, 10 March 2021, https://en.wikipedia.org/wiki/Rosa_Parks.

Sales, Ben. "Meet the Boogaloo Bois, the violent right-wing extremists who (mostly) don't hate the Jews." *Jewish Telegraph Agency,* 5 June 2020, https://www.jta.org/2020/06/05/united-states/meet-the-boogaloo-bois-the-violent-right-wing-extremists-who-mostly-dont-hate-the-jews. Accessed 2021.

Soucheray, Stephanie. "Fauci: Vaccine at least year away, as COVID-19 death toll rises to 9 in Seattle." *CIDRAP News,* 3 Mar. 2020, https://www.cidrap.umn.edu/news-perspective/2020/03/fauci-vaccine-least-year-away-covid-19-death-toll-rises-9-seattle. Accessed 2021.

Taddeo, Sarah. "75-year-old Buffalo man shoved by police speaks out on incident after month in hospital." *USA TODAY,* 31 Aug. 2020, https://www.usatoday.com/story/news/nation/2020/08/31/buffalo-man-martin-gugino-talks-recovery-after-police-shoved-him/3445610001/. Accessed 2021.

Timberg, Craig, et al. "Men wearing Hawaiian shirts and carrying guns add a volatile new element to protests." *The Washington Post,* 4 June 2020, https://www.washingtonpost.com/technology/2020/06/03/white-men-wearings-hawaiian-shirts-carrying-guns-add-volatile-new-element-floyd-protests/. Accessed 2021.

U.S House of Representatives. "Timeline of Trump's Coronavirus Responses." *United States Congressman Lloyd Doggett,*

U.S House of Representatives, 20 Jan. 2021, https://doggett.house.gov/media-center/blog-posts/timeline-trump-s-coronavirus-responses. Accessed 2021.

Vallejo, Justin. "Minneapolis police officer Thomas Lane didn't check George Floyd's 'counterfeit' $20 note." *Independent,* 21 Aug. 2020, https://www.independent.co.uk/news/world/americas/george-floyd-thomas-lane-counterfeit-20-derek-chauvin-a9682781.html. Accessed 2021.

Viglione, Giuliana. "Four ways Trump has meddled in pandemic science- and why it matters." *Nature,* 3 Nov. 2020, https://www.nature.com/articles/d41586-020-03035-4. Accessed 2021.

Woodall, Candy. "George Floyd protests in Pa. being hijacked by white supremacists, state official says." *The Times,* 2 June 2020, https://www.timesonline.com/story/news/local/2020/06/02/george-floyd-protests-in-pa-being-hijacked-by-white-supremacists-state-official-says/112781346/. Accessed 2021.

www.ingramcontent.com/pod-product-compliance
Lightning Source LLC
Chambersburg PA
CBHW020902080526
44589CB00011B/409